PRAISES

It has been a clinical conundrum that when you image [MRI] a cross section of people, there are widespread degenerative changes in the spine but *only a small percentage of those* are suffering from chronic pain. I warmly welcome and encourage the use of these novel strategies in the therapeutic armamentarium in the battle against chronic pain which is still a great drain in productivity and workplace logistics.

Dr. Dheeraj R. Kamalam, MD, board-certified anesthesiologist and interventional pain physician

The road to remission is littered with rabbit holes and dead ends. Thank you, Brajesh, for illuminating the REAL path back to zero pain now. This book will make many lives worth living again.

Edward Glaser, DPM, doctor of podiatric medicine and founder of Sole Supports Inc.

In my time in outpatient clinics and on the wards, I have seen a number of patients who experienced ongoing pain despite the best therapy techniques and modifications. I wish I had considered ALL the biopsychosocial aspects of pain and had access to this book and Brajesh's story sooner. It is a game changer!

Candis Hickman, former occupational therapist, currently a personal branding coach

"A Traffic Signaling Analogy" chapter was so simple to read, and a lightbulb should come on after reading his uplifting story with his end result of NO Pain! I for one will recommend this book for my friends, family and patients to read.

Nanci J. Kersch, LAc., LMT, CT, DTR, HHA, CNA

Hope is the word that I felt throughout reading this book. Hope that is shared by this process and by others who choose to follow.

Marilyn K. Volker, EdD, PhD, sexologist, gender specialist, special needs educator/counselor

Were you told you have to live with the pain? Nothing is less true. If you suffer persistent chronic pain, you'll love this book as you can relate to it AND finally get on a real solution AND discover why everything you've tried so far hasn't worked.

Esther Drost, founder of MagicReset

In this book, Brajesh shows you how to connect to the essence of you, both the good you and the ugly you. And in doing so, he shows that reprogramming embedded old beliefs is possible and that it may be the gateway to ending your years of chronic pain. An entertaining read that delivers incredible amounts of Hope for those in pain.

Leticia Latino, Back2Basics Podcast: Reconnecting to the essence of YOU

Whether it's you or someone close to you suffering with the torment of long-standing pain, this book offers not only hope, but a roadmap to a proven, enduring solution for ending the agony. Buy it, read it, share it!

Clifford Edwards, author of The Forgiveness Handbook: A Simple Guide to Freedom of the Mind and Heart

This book is a must read for those who dream of a pain-free life!

Matilde Machiavello, director at AlmostAlwaysCalm

If you're in pain, read the book to discover the process and test it for yourself.

Ankush Jain, coach, consultant and author of Sweet Sharing: Rediscovering the REAL You

This book provides insight into a psychosomatic technology that we as a culture have yet to master. This book can be a stepping-stone for many to begin their own healing journey.

Rick Marlowe Sostre, executive trainer and coach

Brajesh is a brilliant guide and coach to healing your pain. In this book, he shares his personal pain journey and guides you step by step to rapidly becoming pain-free. Read it and practice it—it's time to live your life fully!

Kathy Zehringer, A Shift Happens

Mr. Singh taught me how to question myself out loud and listen to my out loud answers. Just like he describes in this book. I use this vocal technique if a flare-up threatens to bench me. No pain, I gain.

Sarah, pain-free client

I cancelled my back surgery and I'm now pain-free!

Deborah, pain-free client

Brajesh Singh

The Straw
That Broke the Camel's Back

How I Healed My Back Pain Without Drugs, Surgery,
or Physical Therapy and How You Can Do It Too

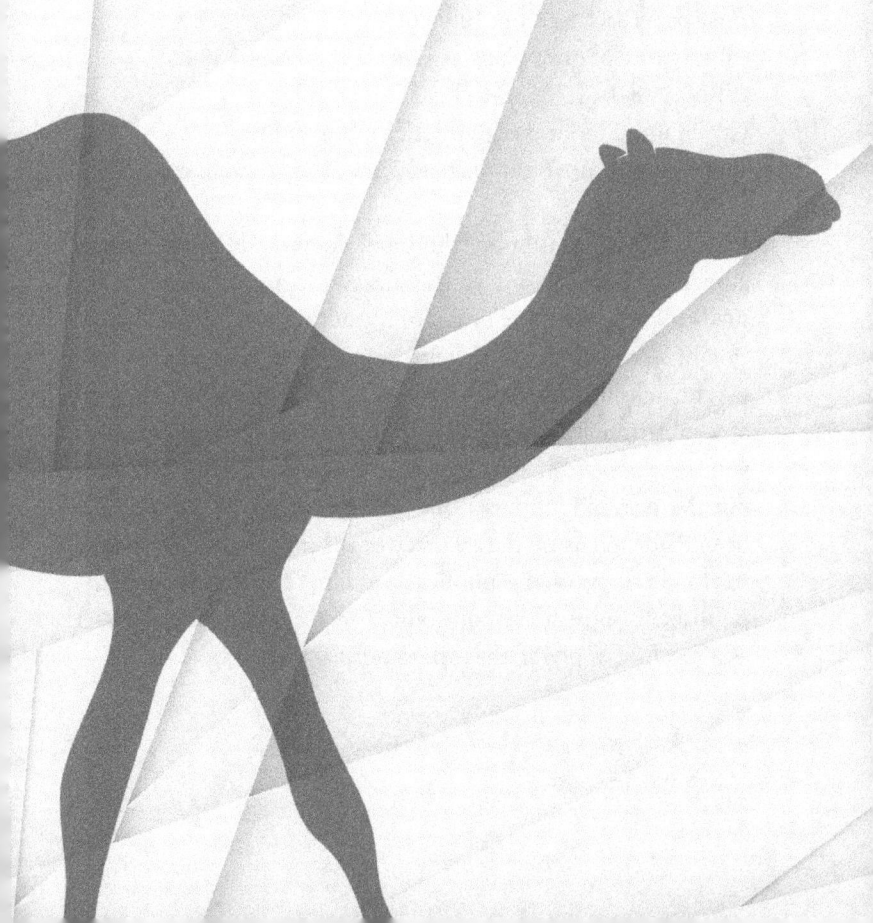

Published by BioPsychoSocialPublishing.com

Copyright © 2022 Brajesh K. Singh. All rights reserved.
No part of this book may be reproduced or transmitted in any form or by any means, electronic or mechanical, including photocopying, recording, or by any information storage or retrieval system, without prior written permission from the publisher.

First paperback edition: July 2022
Library of Congress Control Number: 2022907684
ISBN: 978-1-7376638-0-5
Cover and interior design by Alexandra Andrieş
Photographs copyright unsplash.com, shutterstock.com

Disclaimer: The author of this book does not dispense medical advice or prescribe any technique as a form of treatment for medical problems. The intent of the author is to offer information of a general nature to help the reader in their quest to heal psychologically caused physical pain. The book is not to be used as a substitute for a medical diagnosis or medical treatment. If you are experiencing physical pain, you must see a doctor to rule out the possibility of a serious medical illness. All efforts have been made to ensure the accuracy of the information contained in this book as of the publication date. The author and the publisher assume no responsibility for any actions of the reader as a result of applying these methods.

PREFACE

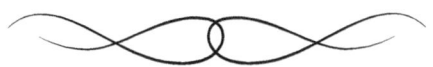

When I talk about chronic pain, I usually get people's attention.

But when I share my story of chronic pain and how I was able to heal myself, that's when people open up and share the story of their own pain. It was as if they needed to hear my story before they could feel what was happening within them.

I see the hope and excitement in their eyes when they realize there is a natural solution to ending their pain. There is a reason that everything they have tried is not working. And it's not their fault.

With that hope and excitement in mind, I have written this book so you too can learn the cause of your pain—*and begin to heal yourself.*

FOREWORD

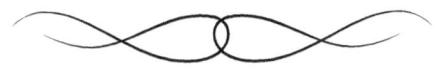

We humans naturally handle positive emotions. Most of us easily process them; it's innate to us. However, processing negative emotions is often an acquired skill. Some people never master it.

Many of us learn that the best way to process or deal with negative emotions is to ignore, suppress, or repress them. This can, and often does, show up in somatic symptoms. Being unaware of our anger and rage and other negative emotions is often the culprit in physiological symptoms. These symptoms can be anything from gastrointestinal problems to chronic physical pain.

Chronic pain usually comes with an incomplete diagnosis and is often blamed on a structural abnormality. However, a more complete and better diagnosis includes the entirety of a person's mental, emotional, and physiological factors.

Once you rule out life-threatening conditions, and when conventional interventions do not eliminate the symptoms, the Zero Pain Now® process is often the best possible methodology. For many people this may be all that you need.

Dr. Hajera Fatima, D.O.

THIS BOOK IS DEDICATED TO ANYONE SUFFERING FROM CHRONIC PAIN.

AND TO MY CLIENTS WHO ARE NOW PAIN-FREE.

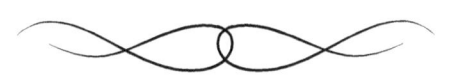

"You think with your body, not only with your brain"
 - *Daniel Kahneman, Nobel Laureate, 2002*

CONTENTS

Praises I
Preface IX
Foreword XI

PART I: AT HOPE'S END 1

Introduction: Year AD 2364 on board the Starship Enterprise 3

1 Billions of People Are in Pain 7
2 Do You Remember When Your Pain Started? 9
3 Can You Touch Your Toes? 13
4 Please Sit Up Straight 15
5 My Dad's Back Pain 17
6 How Do You Take Care of Your Back? 19
7 What "Broke" Your Back? 23
8 How Was Your First Experience With Doctors? 27
9 What Was Your Diagnosis? 31
10 The Book 35
11 Physical Therapy 39
12 Do You Live on the Edge of Pain? 45

PART II: ADRIFT IN PURGATORY 49

13 How Do You Manage Your Life of Pain? 51
14 Yoga 55
15 The McKenzie Method 57
16 Acupuncture 61
17 Swimming 63
18 How Is Your Posture? 69

19	Have Drugs Ever Failed You?	73
20	Do You Feel You Know More Than Your Doctors?	75
21	Did You Get a Second Opinion?	83
22	What Are Your Pain Management Tools?	87
23	Changing the Light Bulb	89
24	How Many Specialists Have You Seen?	91
25	The Last Straw	95
26	Have You Surrendered?	99

PART III: THE HEALING BEGINS 101

27	Can Words Heal You?	103
28	The Placebo and Nocebo Effects	105
29	Trusting the Mind-Body Connection	111
30	A Traffic Signaling Analogy	117
31	The Mistakes I Made	123
32	The Cause	127
33	Understanding Step 2	131
34	The Straw That Broke My Back	133
35	Diversion Pain Syndrome	139
36	Are You a Perfectionist?	143
37	How Do You Know You Are Healed?	149
38	Mike's Back Pain	153
39	Lisa's Neck Pain	155
40	John's Knee Pain	157
41	Carla's Back Pain	159
42	Israel's Back Pain	161
43	Carlos's Undiagnosable Back Pain	163
44	How You Can Heal Yourself	165
45	Final Words	171
	Frequently Asked Questions	175
	Acknowledgements	179
	References	181
	About the Author	185

"The human understanding when it has once adopted an opinion draws all things else to support and agree with it. And though there be a greater number and weight of instances to be found on the other side, yet these it either neglects and despises, or else by some distinction sets aside and rejects."

- *Sir Francis Bacon, AD 1561*

PART I
AT HOPE'S END

INTRODUCTION
YEAR AD 2364 ON BOARD THE STARSHIP ENTERPRISE

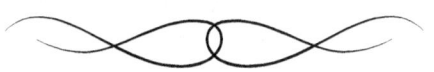

I am a pain sufferer like you. Many years ago I was watching a show on television that included the following dialogue:

"You want to replace his entire spinal column?" asked Dr. Crusher.

"Yes. This'll be the first time it's ever been attempted," replied Dr. Russell.

"No, I'm afraid I can't justify the risk to Worf. We'll have to do with more conventional approaches."

This is a scene from *Star Trek*, one of my favorite shows, where Commander Worf was injured and undergoing spinal surgery.[1]

As I watched a rerun of this episode, it brought tears to my eyes—not because I cared for Commander Worf, but because the scene was speaking to me, telling me I didn't have any hope for my spine, even several hundred years in the future!

I cried, wishing that technology would be available *now* to replace my spine. Why couldn't it be available in the next few years?

After eight years of living with back pain, I had found so many "remedies" that didn't work.

Little did I know that, after suffering for eight years, I was soon to discover a solution to end my pain permanently without drugs, without surgery, and without any physical therapy. And that this solution would allow me to live a normal life and realize that my spine was perfectly normal, just as defective as it was, that there was *nothing wrong* with my spine. I know this sounds contradictory, but I will explain this later in the book.

And there is a very good chance that there is nothing wrong with yours too, or with whatever part of your body that has been labeled with a chronic pain diagnosis.

This is the solution I'm going to share with you in this book to help you get pain-free. It's a solution I learned from Zero Pain Now®. It was so effective at eliminating my chronic pain, and eliminating pain for thousands of others, that I decided to be trained as a certified Zero Pain Now® Master Coach.

Here is what a friend wrote after we had a one-hour phone call about her pain:

> When I mentioned about my upper back pain to Brajesh, I had been suffering from upper back pain due to asthma (or so I thought) for over a year. In that year, my doctor checked for any blood clots, did a full lung-functioning test and various other tests to figure out what was causing the upper back pain. When Brajesh mentioned the Zero Pain Now® theory, I kind of listened to him but didn't pursue

Year AD 2364 on board the Starship Enterprise

it any further. A year later, I was suffering for weeks with upper back pain, and I thought I have nothing to lose by trying this Zero Pain Now® method even though it sounded strange and unbelievable. I had a one-hour phone call with Brajesh and my pain went from worse to less severe, and by the end of our conversation, it was gone. Just like that. It is hard to believe, yet it's true. I still get my upper back pain occasionally but I can heal myself in a matter of minutes.

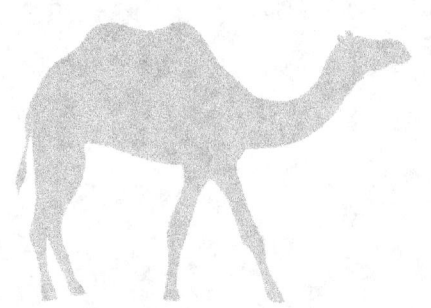

1
BILLIONS OF PEOPLE ARE IN PAIN

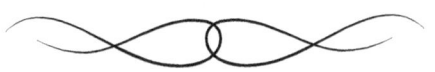

According to a study by Boston University, about 1.5 billion people (or one person in five) in the world suffer from chronic pain right now—recurring pain that lasts longer than a few months.[2] You are reading this book because you are one of them, you are in pain, or you know someone who is in pain and you want a solution. I get it. I've been there. I can help you get better.

While I've used the proven solution described in this book for my back pain, the process of healing applies to many other types of chronic pain, such as:

> Pain in the back, neck, shoulder, sciatic nerve, hip, knee, or foot, migraines, TMJ (temporomandibular joint), whiplash, fibromyalgia, CRPS (Complex Regional Pain Syndrome), herniated disc, bulging disc, spinal stenosis, scoliosis, degenerative disc disease, neuropathy, tendonitis, carpal tunnel syndrome, spondylosis, spondylitis, plantar fasciitis, torn rotator cuff, torn meniscus, osteoarthritis-related pain, bone spurs, undiagnosable pain, and more.

If you are experiencing any one of these, there is more than a 90 percent chance that you can heal yourself, and in this book I will tell you how.

What you've tried isn't working, and it's *not* your fault.

Follow along with my story even though your story may not be the same, your symptoms may not be the same, and your diagnosis may not be the same. If you can *relate to my story of pain,* that's all that matters for you to heal yourself—and you'll find out why. Look at this surprising fact about the cost of chronic pain:

> Chronic pain contributes to an estimated $600 BILLION each year, more than cancer, diabetes, and heart disease COMBINED.
> **National Institutes of Health**

2
DO YOU REMEMBER WHEN YOUR PAIN STARTED?

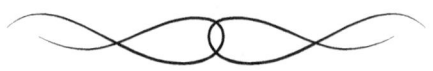

One day your pain started. Whether it was back, jaw, neck, shoulder, knee, hip, or foot pain, or migraines or fibromyalgia or some other pain. Whatever it was, it's now chronic, and whatever you try to do to heal, it keeps returning.

You wonder to yourself:

- What did I do that started it?
- What was the straw that broke the camel's back?
- Or, what was the straw that broke my back?
- And how can I end it?

The saying "the straw that broke the camel's back" describes the seemingly minor or routine action that causes an unpredictably large and sudden reaction because of the cumulative effect of small actions.[3]

Your pain is probably like that. Something small triggers it—perhaps the weather, perhaps driving or playing sports, perhaps sitting down, bending, raising your arm, lifting something, or even just standing up—and you end up in excruciating pain. You want to know what's causing it. You want to know why it happens.

In this book I will give you the answers to the following:

- What started it
- How you can stop it without drugs, surgery, or physical therapy
- How you can stop it by yourself
- How you can heal yourself

This book is about me, but it's really about you too.

This bears repeating: Follow along with my story even though your story, your symptoms, your diagnosis may not be the same. *If you can relate to my story of pain, that's all that matters for you to get better.* I'll tell you why.

Let's begin with my story, which will help you to understand what the cause is of most chronic pain.

One day in 2009 I drove home and parked my car in my garage. It was a new coupe with stiff, tight bucket seats, and while the car was fun to drive, I felt cramped in it each time I drove it. As I opened my car door to get out, it felt like a knife had stabbed me in my lower back. I had excruciating pain, and I couldn't lift my leg to step out of the car.

I had never experienced something like this before, and I couldn't believe this was happening to me. Here I am, sitting in my garage at the age of 37, and I can't even get out of my car. The pain intensified with any movement I made, even taking my hands off the steering wheel.

**Do you remember the first time you
experienced debilitating chronic pain?**

I sat there for 10 minutes in stabbing pain, eyes closed, heart pounding, wondering, What should I do? I'd never heard of this happening to anyone before. Do I call 911? Yell for my neighbor? Start the car and try to drive to someone who could help me?

This was the moment the straw broke the camel's back. This was the start of my eight years of excruciating back pain. Over the previous months my pain had gradually increased whenever I sat in this tight seat and culminated with this debilitating moment when I arrived home that day. For the next eight years I tried everything to heal and get better, but nothing worked.

To understand how I was able to heal myself from my pain, we need to look at back pain and chronic pain like a mystery being solved by Sherlock Holmes—one of my favorite fictional detectives.

I love this phrase from Sherlock Holmes[4]: "Once you eliminate the impossible, whatever remains, no matter how improbable, must be the truth." This book is about eliminating the impossible. This is how we will discover the straw that broke the camel's back. Or my back. Or your back or any part of your body that has chronic pain.

You will see that the solution is easy and simple, and it makes sense once you take this journey with me and see how I was able to eliminate all the false leads at the scene of the crime.

I am an engineer. My job is problem-solving, so you may appreciate the methodical way I will take you through this journey. I am a perfectionist and results focused. The solution in this book is based on results. I design communication networks, complex systems that carry your voice, video, and data instantly from one corner of the world to the other. Your body is also a complex system, carrying messages to every cell in your body, and yes, there are many similarities.

I am one of the lucky many who were able to heal themselves, and now I've been pain-free since 2017. When my pain started, I imagined the pain would go away in a few days. I had no idea it would last eight years.

Like I said, I am one of the lucky ones to have discovered how to heal myself, even though the solution is in plain sight. To see it, however, we have to eliminate the impossible. I've now helped many clients get pain-free—some of whom have been in pain for more than 40 years. *The only thing they wished was that they had been told about this solution earlier.* But this is not a matter of luck, it's a matter of telling the whole world about this solution and changing our understanding about the cause and origin of the majority of noncancer-related chronic pain.

So, whether you've suffered six months or 50 years, you're in the right place, because in this book I am going to show you how you can heal yourself, how to stop all drugs and physical therapy, and without any need for surgery, how you can get back to the way you were before the pain, possibly even better, and live a normal life.

To understand the solution, we need to take a journey back in time, because this is important to learn how to get out of your pain. If you can relate to this journey, you have the best chance of getting out of your pain and back to a life doing everything you've always wanted to do—a life filled with smiles and whatever physical activity you can't do now.

3
CAN YOU TOUCH YOUR TOES?

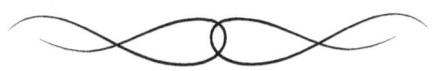

When I was nine years old, I was a chubby, overweight kid. In my physical education class I remember my gym teacher asked us to touch our toes, and my fingers could barely reach below my knees. She was about 40 years old—which is like really old when you're nine—and she said she didn't practice touching her toes when she was young and that was why she has back pain. The message was clear: All of us must be able to touch our toes, otherwise we too will get back pain.

This is where my programming began, where my mind was imprinted with beliefs that really cannot be challenged. Who was I, at nine years old, to question my wise old gym teacher? And what a coincidence that I got my pain when I was close to 40?

From that day onward, I kept trying to touch my toes by lunging down, and eventually I would just be able to touch them with the tips of my fingers. But that was as far as I could get. I was convinced I wasn't flexible enough because I wasn't able to touch my toes like the other students.

> **Do you remember the first time you were told to touch your toes?**

The Straw That Broke the Camel's Back

There are plenty of people who can't touch their toes yet don't have back pain.

4
PLEASE SIT UP STRAIGHT

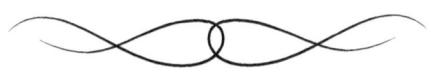

Next I went to history class. History always put me to sleep. I couldn't remember all those dates of battles and who did what and when. So mostly I would slump in my chair and try to fall asleep with my eyes open, hoping the teacher wouldn't notice and wouldn't ask me any questions.

But, of course, I was the perfect example the teacher could use to tell everyone, "Don't slump like Brajesh." The message was that you've got to sit up straight and keep a straight spine, otherwise your spine will be curved.

You might remember this too. "Stop slumping and sit up straight, stick your chest out. You don't want to be seen slumped. After all, image is everything, isn't it?" I didn't challenge it then, and while I'm not advocating slumping now, there are plenty of people who sit up straight and still have back pain.

5
MY DAD'S BACK PAIN

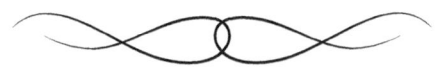

Then, when I was 14, my dad was at the airport, and he lifted his heavy suitcase from the conveyer belt. Something popped in his back and he couldn't walk he was in so much pain. His doctor told him he had a slipped disc and needed emergency surgery. Scared of surgery, my dad decided to stay home and rest. My mother prepared a flat bed made out of wood, and for three days he lay on this hard piece of wood, not moving. Fortunately, after three days his back felt better, and he was able to return to normal activity.

Ever since then he always reminded me to take care of my back. To this day he tells me how he nearly had to have surgery and that he was very lucky he was able to heal from a slipped disc. He says the only solution to a bad back is to lie on a hard bed for three days and not move. When I got my back pain, he reminded me many times that I should do this and I'll be better.

There is now a whole mattress industry out there telling you why a soft mattress is better, or a firm mattress is better. But remember, people slept fine well before such expensive mattresses were ever invented, and you can too. You don't have to sleep in pain anymore.

> **Do you get advice from others about
> how to make your pain better?**

But it's probably unlikely these people are suffering like you, or at least able to relate to you with their ongoing aches and pains.

6
HOW DO YOU TAKE CARE OF YOUR BACK?

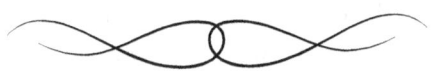

Perhaps you've been told that the back is fragile and must be taken care of. There are so many rules on how to do that. I imagine you have heard most of these: You should stretch your muscles before exercise. Warm up first. Touch your toes. Keep your back straight. Swimming is good for your back. You should strengthen your core so the muscles protect your spine. The correct way to lift is by bending at the knees. A sedentary lifestyle causes back pain. As you get older you get more pain. You should sleep on a firm mattress. A spine once injured does not easily heal. Sports can injure you. And on and on.

Over the years I heard a myriad of different solutions that help to have a good back. For example, the proper way to lift is by bending at the knees. This made little sense to me because growing up in India and Africa, I saw people bending at the waist, hinging their upper body at their hips when they were bending down and working and lifting.

I didn't see anyone lifting from their knees, and the prevalence of back pain is much lower in developing countries than it is in the United States and the Western world.⁵ Wouldn't they have naturally figured out that lifting with bent knees was better? A study in the *Scandinavian Journal of Pain* found no difference between lifting with bent knees and hinging at the hips. Many similar studies have been conducted disputing the prevailing guideline of lifting by bending at the knees.⁶

Neither did the common belief about a sedentary lifestyle leading to back pain sound right to me. I had seen plenty of people sitting all day long, just on the ground, and they didn't have pain, like the man sitting in the picture below. No fancy eight-way adjustable chair that cost $999, either.

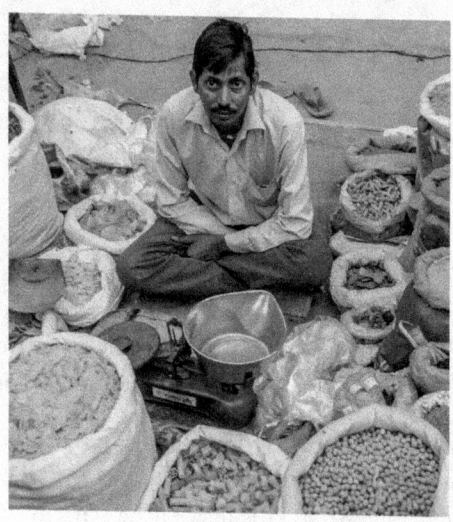

In India there's a special kind of porter at a railway station platform called a coolie. His job is to carry your luggage and get you into the train as fast as possible. I remember that many of these coolies were older men, easily over the age of 50, and they would pick up my suitcase and my dad's suitcase and my mom's suitcase and my brother's suitcase and pile them all on their head and then run faster than we could keep up—and get us into the train on time! Below is a picture of a coolie at work.

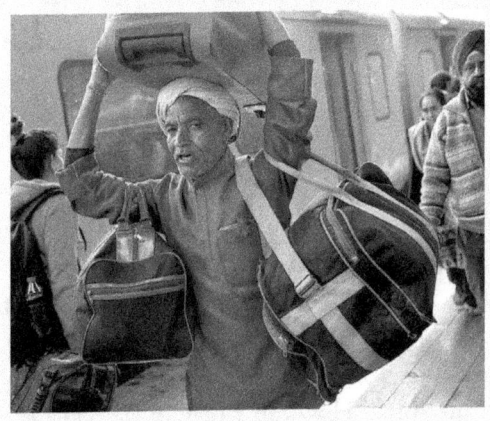

So it was puzzling to me that I was being taught these new ways of sitting and lifting. Wouldn't people have figured this out on their own, especially those that lift every day for their living? And placing weights on our heads is usually an absolute no-no, while this practice is common in developing countries. You have probably seen images of African women carrying jugs of water on their heads.

I've heard messages in the media that a back injury does not heal easily and that the back is fragile. And a conflicting message that doing physical activity keeps your back strong. If the back is so fragile, why would physical activity not injure it? How do circus contortionists and Cirque du Soleil performers do their amazing body movements?

I always admired dancers, how they could spin and run and lift and do all these amazing movements with their bodies well into old age. Our backs must be much stronger than we think they are, and yet there was all this conflicting messaging coming at me about how fragile it is.

Chronic pain with professional athletes is common. It is estimated that about 50 percent of National Football League (NFL) players are in pain, promoting the idea that we can get chronically injured in sports.[7] Here's what one of the greatest tennis players of all time, Andre Agassi, wrote:

> When the nerves test their cramped quarters, they send out distress signals, a pain runs up and down my leg that makes me suck in my breath and speak in tongues.... I grab my back. It grabs me. I feel as if someone snuck in during the night and attached one of those antitheft steering wheel locks to my spine. How can I play in the US Open with the club on my spine? Will the last match of my career be a forfeit?[8]

Andre Agassi won the US Open in 2006 on the same day described above. How is that possible?

By the age of 37 I was filled with a lot of information about what causes back pain.

What beliefs do you have about your chronic pain?

7
WHAT "BROKE" YOUR BACK?

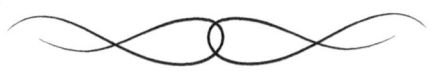

Let's return to me sitting in my car in pain.

My story begins in 2009 when there was a financial crisis, the crash of the housing market and the bursting of the telecom bubble. Because of this and other factors, the company I worked for (my first job, in fact) for the last 15 years declared Chapter 11 bankruptcy. More than 50,000 people lost their jobs. Somehow I survived the layoffs, but I lost almost all my retirement savings. Our office buildings were sold off, and we were told to start working from home to save money.

Grateful for still having my job and worried that things could get worse, I started working for longer periods, spending sometimes 14 hours a day or more sitting at my desk and working away on my computer.

I had also recently bought a new car, a sports coupe with tight bucket seats.

About three months after buying my new car, I started experiencing low-back pain every time I would get out of the car—a kind of a stiff grinding feeling in my lower back. I blamed it on the tight bucket seats, which were far less comfortable than my old sedan. I figured it would be some time before I would get used to the new seats.

Then one day I came home and parked in my garage. When I opened my car door, I felt an excruciating pain like a knife stabbing me in the back. Any little movement intensified the pain. There I was, sitting in my garage and I couldn't even get out of my car.

I sat there for ten minutes wondering what to do. I realized there was only one way to get out of the car. So I opened the door wider and tilted my body sideways until I fell partway out. Using my hands almost in a wheelbarrow style, I crawled completely out and lay on my garage floor crying in pain.

Having accomplished getting out of my car, I felt a little better and was able to hobble into my house, lie down, and get some rest while wondering what was going on with me.

I was afraid to get back in my car. What if that happened again? It was the car seat that was causing my back pain. I Googled the model of my car and, sure enough, about 20 other people had posted similar complaints on a car forum that their back pain had increased after buying this particular car. I was angry and wanted to sue the manufacturer. I even called them and filed a complaint.

At the young age of 37 I was now disabled and scared. I was hardly able to move. I called a friend to ask her to bring me some groceries. I called my brother, who came to assist me for a few weeks and drive me around and help me get back on my feet, literally.

What was new to me was how invisible my illness was. Friends and family would come up to me as if I were normal, and only when I told them I was in pain would they look at me and wonder how I could be in pain when I looked so normal. And I couldn't explain how I injured my back. Everyone asked, "What happened?" I didn't play sports. I didn't catch a baby falling out of a burning building. I didn't have an accident or injury. I hadn't lifted a heavy load. What was the cause of this injury to my back?

What "broke" *your* back?

I hated this question. I wished I could have given a better and more interesting and believable answer. Perhaps yours was an injury or an accident. The only answer I could give was that it was the tough and uncomfortable car seat. And my sedentary lifestyle, especially working long hours just sitting at home. People would nod at me understandingly, reinforcing the belief in me that it was true, and probably to themselves it was true.

Well, I thought, whatever it is, doctors will tell me. So I sought medical attention.

8
HOW WAS YOUR FIRST EXPERIENCE WITH DOCTORS?

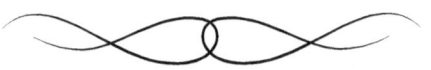

If you've experienced the same sudden onset of chronic pain as me, you might be able to relate how life changes in one day. Suddenly I was unable to do something as simple as brushing my teeth. I experienced so much pain while bending forward that I had to lean against the bathroom counter.

On the other hand, you might not even be able to remember a time without pain.

I made an appointment at one of the best hospitals in the world, the Cleveland Clinic. I assumed the doctor would do some careful diagnostics, ask me a lot of detailed questions, and be able to fix whatever was happening to me. At this point, I didn't know what chronic pain was.

However, as might have been your experience, apparently I was just another number. I was seen for about five minutes, and then I was asked if I wanted an injection.

Injection? I didn't even know what that meant. I learned later that injections help get rid of the pain. The doctor assumed

I knew what he was talking about, so he didn't even bother to explain what an injection was. After a brief analysis in which he asked me where my pain was, he said, "Lower back? Oh, OK. We need to schedule an MRI, and then you can go home."

That's it?

My last three weeks I've been hobbling around like a 90-year-old, and you spend five minutes with me, offer me an injection, and then tell me to get an MRI? That's how advanced medical science has become? Nothing about my car or my chair or my habits? Or a detailed physical examination of my back? Nothing about reporting this car manufacturer to OSHA or some consumer organization?[9]

Medical science can see the DNA of our cells. We can edit genes. We can do pinpoint robotic surgery. We can photograph the atom. Insert a stent into the heart through the wrist. We can even develop a Covid vaccine in just 2 days.[10] But for my back pain, you ask me if I want an injection?

At that time I wasn't consciously aware of these thoughts, but I knew something wasn't right with the way I was being treated. I was shuffled out of the doctor's office and the next patient was brought in.

Was your first visit with your doctor brief and confusing?

When I came home, my head was spinning. My whole world had turned upside down, and the doctor had spent only five minutes with me as if this happens to people every day? At one of the top hospitals in the world? Doesn't he realize I'm disabled? What if I'm stuck with this for the rest of my life?

I went to my MRI appointment, and I had to remove all metal in preparation for the MRI. I was inserted into a narrow white tube, wearing just a hospital gown, and a noise began that sounded like laser guns firing in a *Star Wars* movie. I was in so much pain and fear of what the MRI machine would detect. As it was noisily scanning me, I was in pain lying there wondering what was happening to me.

9
WHAT WAS YOUR DIAGNOSIS?

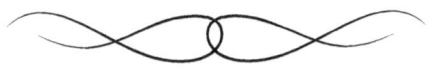

I returned to the doctor to review my MRI results, and I tried to tell him exactly where my pain was so he could use this information to determine which muscle or nerve or bone was creating the pain so he could fix it. However, the doctor didn't seem interested at all in my pointing out where my pain was. He just gave me a glance and continued to look at his papers.

He examined my MRI and showed me the damages in my spine. In my lumbar, I had herniated discs, four degenerated discs, some stenosis, and multiple schmorl's nodes, which is where the disc protrudes into the spinal vertebrae. When I saw that, I had goose pimples all over my body from fear and despair. That image is still burned into my mind today.

How did you feel when you first received your diagnosis?

Today I understand that a diagnosis is simply a way for the medical world to categorize what you have. It's a bucket they put you in. They use it to simplify their communications. A diagnosis is just a classification. It does not mean it is real. It doesn't even mean that they know what it is. It's just a classification.

But to me, hearing the diagnosis was terrifying. These technical medical words were completely new to me. And I had not just one but a list of words I hadn't heard before, nor did I know how to pronounce some of them without seeing them written down.

The doctor told me I had a spine of a 60-year-old. I asked him why that had happened, and he shrugged his shoulders and said, "I don't know. For some people it just happens."

At this point the doctor said some things I didn't understand until many years later.

"Mr. Singh, there are many people with these kinds of structural defects in their spine, and some people experience pain and some people don't, and medical science doesn't have an answer for it. For some people it goes away, and for some people it doesn't go away."

I wish I had paid more attention to what he said. Maybe you've been told something similar. One study reported in *The New England Journal of Medicine* involved 98 people with *no* pain who were given an MRI.[11] It turned out that 66 percent of them had bulging discs and herniated discs. You can find many more studies like this.

> 98 People Studied With No Pain
> 66% Had Bulging Discs and Herniated Discs
> **New England Journal Of Medicine**

The doctor continued, "I can do injections every six months to keep away the pain, or I can recommend some physical therapy to strengthen your core as that seems to help some people with back pain."

I didn't know what to say. I was hoping he was going to make me feel better. I still didn't even know what an injection was, and I was too afraid to ask. I didn't want an injection in my spine.

He went on. "Normal discs have the consistency of jelly beans. Degenerated discs have the consistency of toothpaste. These four dark ones in your spine are degenerated."

Why was he smiling when he was telling me this? I don't think he realized the impact this diagnosis had on me.

The images of my MRI kept replaying in my mind. My disc protruding into the vertebrae. The four black degenerated discs. The herniated discs. I was imagining pain with each step I took, having the back of a 60-year-old, and I began to be afraid of exerting myself physically in any way, like running, climbing several flights of stairs, or playing any active sports. At that moment, I took on the belief that my back is broken, that it is fragile and old and I might not recover. This belief was completely in line with everything I had learned from my childhood. I believed it.

Do you recall the moment when you accepted your diagnosis?

Again the session with him was very short, and I felt angry that my life was turned upside down and all he could do was spend a few minutes with me, give me a list of some technical words I had never heard before, and not even look at my body to see where the pain was or try to figure out what was causing the pain. It was almost as if he didn't know and didn't seem to care. In retrospect, he did care, but I would only understand this later.

Was your experience with doctors similar to this?

I say all this after the fact, but mostly while I was in the doctor's office, my head was foggy and I was unable to think straight. If you've been in chronic pain, I suspect you'll know exactly what I mean. And you've probably been treated similarly.

When I was about to walk out, the doctor looked at me and recommended a book. He said some people get better after reading this book, adding that there might be a mind-body connection to my pain.

"Everyone thinks of changing the world, but no one thinks of changing himself."

- Leo Tolstoy

10
THE BOOK

I returned home and began to Google as much as I could about back pain, searching for the new words on my list of diagnoses from the doctor. The more I searched, the worse I felt. There was so much to read, and yet it gave me no hope, just a lot more medical terms, uncertainty, and a feeling of doom seeing the countless number of people in pain with my diagnoses. I imagine you've done that search for your diagnosis too.

back pain solutions

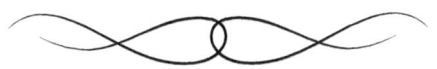

About 529,000,000 results (1.36 seconds)

I found millions and millions of articles, and millions and millions of reasons, and millions and millions of solutions to the point where I felt so overwhelmed that I cried. Take a look. Five hundred million hits on Google and probably an even higher count by the time you read this book.

I ordered the book the doctor recommended: *Healing Back Pain: The Mind-Body Connection* by Dr. John Sarno.[12] I began to read it, expecting it to be a step-by-step explanation of my pain. But instead it was a strange book that connected stress and tension to my pain.

About halfway into it was a picture of an eye and the mind and an explosion of pain. I felt furious. The picture looked like it was hand drawn by a child. I wondered how such a nonscientific book could possibly be considered to help with back pain, and I threw it in the trash. The pain is real, it's not in my head!

I was now disillusioned with the medical system and felt helpless and insecure about my future. Only later did I understand why I was being treated this way, and you will see why too.

When there is a problem in engineering, you narrow it down, identify the issue, and solve it. Engaging my engineering mind, I told myself I would figure this out and find out what is not right with me. I will find the straw that broke my back. My goal wasn't to rule out the impossible, but that's how it went.

Engineers are essentially detectives. When something is broken, we take a step-by-step methodical approach to determine the root cause of the problem. Once the root cause is determined and corrected, the problem instantly fixes itself.

Remember, once the root cause is found and corrected, the problem *instantly disappears.*

And so began eight years of experimentation on myself to figure out this mystery of how this pain began. And finally, after eight years, I confess that I gave up. No, don't stop reading! It was only when I gave up that the answer became obvious to me, and that's where I want to take you with this book. When

I had investigated everything and failed to find answers, all that remained was the truth. However, if I had known initially that I would end up doing these experiments for the next eight years, I never would have done it! I want to save you time so you don't have to search in vain like I did and instead get pain-free quickly.

I kept thinking that tomorrow I'll be better, tomorrow I'll be better, tomorrow this will be over. But as sure as you're reading this book, that isn't how it goes, is it?

You're probably trying new solutions frequently too. And maybe you've been trying for years.

> **Are there days you wake up and wonder:**
> **Will I be able to function today?**

How many times will you need to rest or take a break? Will you be able to fulfill all your obligations, or will you make an excuse—perhaps call in sick to work—or lie to someone without telling them you are in pain? And perhaps sit in the shame that they would not understand even if you told them the truth. I've been there. Stay with me, there is a solution.

11
PHYSICAL THERAPY

I sent my dad my MRI, and he showed it to his physician. He called me about an hour later and said that a surgeon had seen my MRI and told him that I needed to have surgery right away, that my spine was completely messed up. This scared me even more. My dad can be very determined, and he kept insisting that I fly to where he was and see his surgeon.

There was no way I was going to have surgery on my back, and I'm glad I didn't choose that option. Did you know that back surgeries have only a 35 percent success rate?[13]

> Back Surgery
> 35% Success Rate
> **National Institutes of Health**

I decided to take up the physical therapy suggested by my doctor. I didn't want to take any drugs; I don't like adding chemicals to my body. I had been living a sedentary lifestyle and sitting on my tight bucket car seat—that must be reason for my pain. I would strengthen my muscles, convinced that soon the pain would be gone!

Little did I know how wrong I was.

And thus began my journey toward healing with physical therapy. Since the doctors had spent no more than a few minutes with me, I imagined that the physical therapist would know the issue and give me much more detail on what was causing my pain.

So you can imagine my surprise when I walked into my physical therapy session and they looked at my referral and said, "Lower back pain?" Then, after about five minutes of doing a few tests with me to see how much I could push with my hands and legs—nothing about where the pain was or how it felt—they prescribed about five different exercises for me to do. I spent more time filling out their forms with my insurance information and health history than they did in looking at my pain.

> **How much time did the specialist spend examining your symptoms?**

Again my mind began to feel dizzy, and I'm only able to write this after recalling it years later. I wondered, How do they know what's wrong with me? How did they diagnose me so fast? What if the exercises they taught me are not the ones that will help me?

I was expecting them to narrow down the exact muscle that was causing me pain, the exact bone that was out of alignment, the exact nerve that wasn't functioning properly, or the exact structure that needed to be corrected. This is how we examine a problem in engineering.

Physical Therapy

But they never even asked me where the pain was, how it comes about, when it comes about, what things I can't do, and what things I can do. Or even what I want to be able to do. Yet at that time these questions didn't occur to me. All I knew was that something wasn't right with the way they were funneling me through the system with a five-minute interview and telling me to do all these things without telling me why they would help me get better, or even telling me more details about what was wrong.

Since there was no visible injury, what if they thought I was making it up? I'm sure I would have received more empathy and attention if my injury were visible.

I did what they were telling me. I asked a lot of questions. For every exercise they told me to practice, I would ask, "Which muscle is this exercising? Which bone is this connected to? What nerve?"

I realized I was irritating them because no one asked so many questions. I insisted that the senior physical therapist explain to me why I was doing all these exercises. They were not used to such patients, and the senior therapist curtly told me: "Mr. Singh, your body is weak and it works as a system. You need to strengthen all of it so your muscles can support your structure."

Have you been given such an explanation? I'm sure you have. It's absolutely believable.

This is what I call an irrefutable explanation. It's the explanation you cannot dispute, you cannot prove them wrong, you cannot say it's not true, yet somewhere deep inside you know it's not the right answer. And my physical therapist was also frustrated. If he had a good answer for me, why would he be frustrated?

In engineering you go to the part that's broken and fix that part. Once you fix that part, all the other parts start working. You don't go around fixing all the other parts and hope that the broken part fixes itself. If you have a flat tire, you don't inflate all the other tires hoping the flat tire will unflatten itself, do you? That might work to get you to a repair shop, but it's just a workaround; eventually you have to fix the flat.

But how was I to explain this to the experts? I was in pain and in their hands. When this was happening, all I knew was something wasn't right and I couldn't put my finger on it. In that moment I trusted that they knew what they were doing.

How is it that one fine day my entire body becomes weak? Yes, it's true I had been sitting 14 hours a day and driving a lot in my new car, but I was still young and could walk and climb stairs. It wasn't logical that suddenly one day all my muscles started to become weak and couldn't support one area of my back. It just didn't make any sense.

Another thing that didn't make sense was that sometimes I would have a different physical therapist, and the new therapist would give me new exercises to do. I would ask, "Why am I doing these different exercises," and I would get that look of a teacher staring at a child who had asked a dumb question.

I was in a system that acted like a machine. There were no explanations, just attendants instructing me on what to do and keeping the machine moving. By the way, I love physical therapists. They are wonderful people who help anyone that is injured and needs rehabilitation, for example, from an accident. I was just not a good fit for them.

Are you in the medical machine of pain management?

As an aside, you might have heard that younger and younger people are now getting back pain and other chronic pains. You might be one of them reading this book. I've heard of several teens with back pain. It's unlikely that back pain is a structural or aging issue when younger people are starting to experience it. A study listed on the National Institutes of Health website shows that the prevalence of low-back pain by the age of 20 was up by 80 percent in 2011.[14] Below are two examples from a Reddit group I follow, where there are hundreds of posts of teenagers in pain. Similar posts are present on Discord servers and Facebook groups.

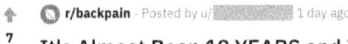

It's Almost Been 10 YEARS and I cannot take it anymore

Since I was 16 I've had intense sciatica pain. All the way from my lower back till my toes. I've tried physiotherapy, Chiropracters, hell even gotten a MRI and according to my doctor nothing showed up in it. (although I genuinely think m

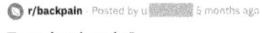

Teen back pain?

Hi I'm an 18 year old female who's been having back pain for about 2 years now. I went to a docto and they did an x-ray and said nothing was wrong and just sent me to physical therapy which didr help. My pain is constant but it is worse some days than others, it's mainly my lower back and it fe like my spine is stiff and compressed, it's so painful and it's affecting my quality of life. I don't knov

A new term for youngsters in chronic pain has emerged—they call themselves spoonies. I'm saddened at seeing these posts, and even more that they too are being put through the same system I went through.

Without being able to express any of this, but knowing that something wasn't right, I put my best foot forward in physical therapy. I came regularly for every appointment. I did every one of the exercises as instructed by my physical therapist. I drew my own pictures of the exercises to make sure I was doing them correctly. My pain became less; it was about a 3 out of 10, and I was able to start taking care of my basic needs in life.

But I was still living on the edge of pain.

12
DO YOU LIVE ON THE EDGE OF PAIN?

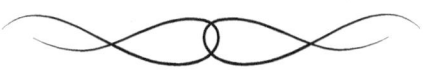

Living on the edge of pain means that if I were to do any increased activity, it would trigger my back into excruciating pain. I would immediately have to lie down in bed for at least a day. Then, the next day I would be able to slowly walk around and just feed and wash myself. On the third day I could sit at a desk and read or watch TV while doing my basic activities. It would take about three weeks before the pain would be down to level 3 again, and then I could live life at 30 percent. So, while the pain was down to level 3, I was actually living life in slow motion. Putting it another way, I was living at a physical ability of a 3 out of 10.

What is your average level of physical ability?

I still couldn't carry more than half a gallon of milk, and vacuuming or cleaning my house took me about three times longer than it used to because I would do things slowly and with the lightest load possible, or spread things out over days instead of cleaning everything all at once.

The Straw That Broke the Camel's Back

To give you an idea of the kind of pain I was experiencing, when I went to the grocery store, I couldn't use a grocery cart because the effort needed to steer it would trigger my back to spasm. The same occurred when brushing my teeth; I had to lean with one hand on the counter. And again when stirring a pot while cooking. I could no longer cook chicken curry, one of my favorite dishes, which can take a lot of stirring during the preparation. I couldn't sleep on my side or get out of bed without rolling and propping myself up on my elbow. And the list goes on and on—anything that required adjusting the positions of my body so my pain wouldn't flare up.

So I would usually buy just enough light groceries that I could carry in my hands to the checkout counter. I couldn't even carry a handbasket because that would put weight on one side of my body and cause the muscle to spasm that results in excruciating pain. I would eat mostly prepared foods and cook simple things like rice.

After experiencing that sitting in my car seat triggered my pain, now I found that I couldn't sit on any chair that had a hard or moving surface, or a chair that didn't have a backrest. When I would go to restaurants, I would sit on all the different chairs they had until I found the one that aggravated my back the least, and then ask the staff if I could move that chair to my table. I couldn't sit on a bar stool or my back would spasm almost immediately. My close friends understood this and were often supportive.

I didn't dare go on a roller coaster for fear of what would happen if my back spasmed in the middle of the upside-down loop. I was unable to go to movie theaters because the chairs in movie theaters recline once you sit on them, and this reclining motion would trigger pain.

The hardest part of living like this was that at times other people didn't understand. Once, some friends insisted that I go with them to a movie. They told me that I would be fine, that the seats were very comfortable. I felt embarrassed that I couldn't even go to a movie theater, so I went with them. But halfway through the movie my pain became so excruciating I had to walk out. I wondered, *What was the straw that broke my back this time?*

Rather than apologizing for coaxing me to go to the theater, they all laughed and said I missed a good movie. I realized they had no idea what I was going through. Very few people do. Can you relate to this? That others can't relate to you and they just laugh?

I could walk but I couldn't run. Sometimes when people would walk fast, I wasn't able to keep up, so they would look at me and say, "Come on, can't you walk faster?" And no matter what I said, they would just laugh and say, "You're being lazy" or "Just keep up, you can do it."

I once saw some breaking news about an active shooter in a mall, with footage showing frenzied shoppers running out of the mall. I watched, terrified, because I started to imagine that if I was ever in such an emergency situation, how would I be able to run away given my back pain? It was easy for me to get caught up in such nightmare scenarios and bring down my usual cheerfulness about life. One of my clients said it perfectly: "I just avoided doing anything that caused me pain."

What activities do you avoid doing because of your pain?

My back pain was like an invisible illness. From the outside I looked fine. But on the inside I was in constant pain, constantly at the edge of a spasm. I would go to a party or birthday celebration, and people would be dancing. But of course dancing triggered my pain, so I would just watch and tap my feet. My friends would pull me onto the dance floor insisting that "dancing is good for you" or telling me not to be so introverted and to have a good time. I would have to extricate myself and go sit down. I would usually end up having a flare-up of my pain.

Even though I didn't know how to dance, this was one of the things I missed not being able to do, to just loosen up and have fun on the dance floor. I had given up dancing in this lifetime—or so I thought.

After six weeks of physical therapy my core was stronger, and I was expecting all my pain to be gone. But this was far from the case. Yes, I was able to manage the pain, but I was still living on a trigger edge. Certain activities were completely out of my scope.

"People travel to wonder at the height of mountains, at the huge waves of the sea, at the long courses of rivers, at the vast compass of the ocean, at the circular motion of the stars; and yet they pass by themselves without wondering."

- Saint Augustine, AD 354

PART II
ADRIFT IN PUGATORY

13
HOW DO YOU MANAGE YOUR LIFE OF PAIN?

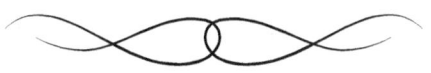

When they discharged me from physical therapy after six weeks, I asked them "Why is the pain still there? If my muscles are now stronger, why hasn't the pain gone?" They said I needed to continue the physical therapy exercises at home for probably at least three more months. I'm sure they were happy they could check off one more client who would not be irritating them with unanswerable questions anymore.

Again, this answer made no sense to me. And again, how could I dispute this answer? I don't think they knew how to answer it, and this was probably the standard answer they give to everyone.

Physical therapists are wonderful at helping people with acute pain or an injury to get back on their feet. At the time I didn't realize they couldn't help me because I was suffering from chronic pain.

Living at 30 percent of what I was able to do before was hardly satisfactory. I couldn't lift things more than a few pounds. I couldn't participate in outdoor activities and games or even ride a bicycle. On especially painful days I would wear a back brace just to get my daily chores done.

I bought a memory foam car seat to put on top of my hard bucket seat, and this helped to stop the seat from triggering my spasm. I could drive for about half an hour without any increase in pain.

Continuing my exercises was definitely not working for me, even though I got stronger and stronger, lifting more weights and doing more exercises than what was originally required of me. I was hoping I could get my body to a level of strength where I would no longer have pain. But what was really happening was that my pain was getting even worse because my muscles were now stronger. I would do exercises, gain strength, feel a lot of confidence that this was helping my pain, only to sit on an uncomfortable chair and immediately spasm and have my pain triggered, which was now even more painful than before because I was stronger.

When I called the physical therapist to ask why this was happening, I was told that I needed to do the exercises exactly as described and that I probably wasn't doing them right or lifting correctly. I may need to come back in and learn how to do them again.

This made no sense. Not only was I highly motivated to get better, but I'm a perfectionist. I paid close attention to how the exercises were done, and even found videos of those exercises on YouTube to match them. It was highly unlikely that I was doing them incorrectly. I don't think they really knew why it wasn't working either, so they gave their standard answer.

What made it worse was that for every exercise I found on YouTube, I found another video saying why I shouldn't do that exercise. Nothing was consistent. There were contradictions everywhere I looked.

I bought a balance ball, a large inflated rubber ball that you can sit on to do various exercises for your back. I also bought heat pads and ice pads and a TENS (transcutaneous electrical nerve stimulation) machine to use at home, just like they used at the physical therapist's office. This machine has electrodes that stick to your skin and generate electric shocks to stimulate the muscles underneath. I bought massager devices and Epsom salts for warm baths. I was able to mostly replicate the physical therapy environment at home.

Something that didn't make sense was that no one could definitively tell me whether I should use heat or ice to relieve the pain. Both seemed to work, but not consistently, sometimes heat would work and sometimes ice. Sometimes the TENS machine would work, and sometimes I would stimulate my muscles for a full hour with no reduction in the pain. Sometimes the Epsom salt baths would work, and sometimes they wouldn't.

Do you experience contradictions with your pain management methods?

I walked around carrying a back cushion with me wherever I went. I would use it on every uncomfortable seat. If I forgot my cushion, I would usually just stand. I sometimes wondered who designed such uncomfortable seats, especially on trains, buses, and airplanes. I dreamed of becoming a seat designer for ergonomic furniture so people in pain would have relief.

My self-confidence dropped within a few years of being in pain. I was limited in where I could meet people and what activities I could participate in. I was afraid of exerting myself beyond anything except walking in case I would trigger my pain.

I was limited in how often I could be sexual for fear that my pain would return. Being in chronic pain is a downward spiral, and its effects snowball into one another, leading to depression and more pain.

What is dating and romance like with your chronic pain?

I often canceled dates and social events because of my pain. I lost interest in dating and developed low self-esteem.

14
YOGA

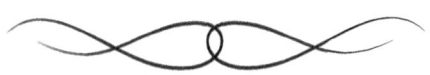

A close friend is a yoga instructor. She told me, "Brajesh, yoga is excellent for the back. And you're Indian, so you already know that. You should come to my class. It will help with your back pain." She was right. I do know that yoga is good for a long life.

"Thanks, Lily, but I'm afraid if I do the wrong movement, I'll hurt myself. You know, I'll be doing the downward dog pose, and I'll stay stuck like a dog."

She laughed. "Don't worry, I teach gentle yoga. It's more meditative with small gentle movements. You'll be fine, and you'll get great healing benefits from it."

"OK, I'll try it."

So I showed up at her yoga class. The participants sat on chairs, with soothing music playing in the background. All we had to do was lift one foot off the ground and straighten the leg out in front of us. I thought, I should be able to do this. I lifted my left leg up slowly. Immediately my muscle spasmed. Ouch! *What was the straw that broke my back this time?* I winced in pain while my friend smiled at me, and her smile was saying, "Isn't this wonderful? Don't you feel better?"

My wince should have indicated "No, I don't."

I left the class and later made up an excuse, saying I had an emergency. How could I explain to my friend that I had spasmed my muscle in just one minute of her gentle yoga class? I didn't even understand that myself. *Isn't yoga supposed to be good for my back?* What's wrong with me?

Since that day I often get told that I should do yoga, and I politely decline. The belief that yoga helps with back pain is as ingrained as the notion that mice like cheese. In fact, mice prefer peanut butter; cheese is just a belief from the cartoons.

15
THE MCKENZIE METHOD

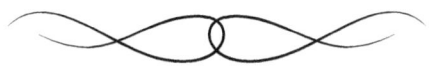

I began to look for other ways to get better. While searching online, I found a remedy called the McKenzie Method. It was discovered accidentally by a physical therapist who saw a patient heal rapidly by doing a certain movement. Excited by the prospect of getting my life back in a short amount of time, I bought a book on the McKenzie Method and immediately began to read about how to implement it.

The McKenzie Method requires you to do a few simple exercises for three minutes every day to keep the pain away. Until now I had been spending hours a day managing my pain. The first day I did the McKenzie Method exercises I felt noticeably better and was excited that this might be the solution I had been looking for.

For about three days I felt great, like I used to feel before I was in pain, and I was confident that I was going to get better. I even ordered the McKenzie cushion and other recommended accessories—some of which I still have today. But on the fourth day, while doing the exercises, I felt a sudden spasm followed by sharp debilitating pain in my lower back muscle. *Oh no! What was the straw that broke my back this time?*

As I have mentioned before, once my muscle spasms, it takes about three weeks before it gets better. So for the next three days I pretty much had to lie in bed and order takeout food to be delivered to me because I couldn't even cook or drive due to the pain.

How long are you out for after a flare-up?

This was the price I paid for every new remedy I tried: I would read about something new, I would be optimistic that it would work, I would try it and it would seem to provide some improvement, but just when I was feeling good about it, my muscle would spasm.

You can imagine what this did to my self-esteem and optimism. The more I would try something, the more the pain would return and the less I would want to try anything else, especially because the pain would last for three weeks. This was the price of trying new things—a cyclical downward spiral. Perhaps you can relate to this too.

This is where family and friends are not helpful at all, because they continually tell you to try new things. They don't understand that there is a price for trying something new. And they tell you to stick to the method for months and not simply try it for a short period of time.

There's a whole business model for back pain built around this idea of long-term care: statements like "It takes at least six sessions to notice any improvement," or "It's like a dental plan. It's preventative care, you must do this for the rest of your life," and so on.

It's possible you're at this stage right now, where you've tried so many new things that you don't like getting your hopes up just to be inevitably disappointed. You may now have become averse to trying new things and instead prefer to play it safe by avoiding doing anything that triggers your pain. Maybe you have accepted just living a subdued life at 30 percent of your capabilities. I was just getting started in trying solution after solution.

How many solutions have you tried to heal yourself?

Even without success, I was too scared to *stop* my physical therapy routine for fear that my pain would get worse. So I kept following it every day—at least two hours of stretching, warming up, doing the prescribed exercises, applying a hot pack, and then cooling down. Two hours of my daily life that was lost in managing my pain.

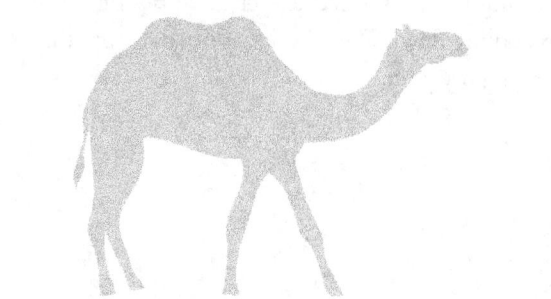

16
ACUPUNCTURE

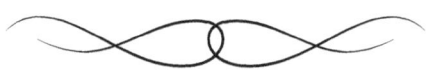

Into my fifth year of pain, I finally acknowledged that what I had was a chronic condition and that I wasn't getting better. A friend of mine pointed me to an acupuncturist. He said she was one of the best, and every few months he visited her for treatments related to conditions other than pain.

I'm skeptical of needles poking me, so I had been avoiding acupuncture even though I had heard of it before. One day I was stuck in traffic for an hour—sitting twice as long as the half hour it took to exacerbate my back pain. I started getting high levels of pain again, so I finally decided to try acupuncture.

I arrived at the clinic and was welcomed into a calming Feng Shui environment with soft music and the gurgling sounds of flowing water. The acupuncturist was friendly, and I lay down and had needles poked in my feet, legs, and lower back. The overall experience was pleasant, and I felt relaxed and rejuvenated.

When I left the clinic, I was afraid to believe that maybe I had finally found the answer. The needles energized my nerves; maybe it was my flow of nervous energy that was causing blockages in my system and now they were clear.

The Straw That Broke the Camel's Back

A few days later I sat on a barstool while chatting with a friend. When I stood up, I felt a little tingling in my lower back. No, I said to myself, I'm healed now. But the tingling turned into a tug, and all of a sudden my muscle spasmed to an excruciating pain. Not again! *What was the straw that broke my back this time?* My friend had to help me get to my car. I decided to give up on acupuncture.

17
SWIMMING

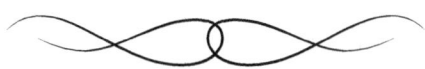

The most common thing people say about swimming is that it exercises every muscle in the body, and the next most common thing is that it's very good for your back. I don't think I can find a single person who would tell me otherwise. It's a commonly known fact that swimming is good for your back, right? Perhaps you have tried swimming too.

I learned to swim when I was seven years old, and I love swimming. But I had stopped swimming after high school.

After giving up physical therapy and the McKenzie Method, and then yoga and acupuncture, I realized I should take up swimming again because "everyone knows" that swimming is one of the best things for your back. So I started to swim laps at my community pool. As I swam I could feel the pain in my back, but I pushed on because I knew that swimming would help me.

The first day I was able to swim four lengths of the pool before I felt tired and exhausted. I came out of the pool feeling stronger muscles. It seemed to be working. Why hadn't I done this sooner? However, the next day my pain returned. I thought to myself that maybe it takes a few weeks before swimming starts to make a difference.

So I went back swimming again.

I was able to increase slowly from four to 20 lengths over several persistent weeks. As I progressed in my swimming, I felt my core muscles getting stronger and tighter. My breathing improved as did my overall stamina. But exactly the same thing happened as in physical therapy. The day after the swimming, the pain would return, and since my muscles were getting stronger, the pain would also get stronger.

When I would discuss this with friends, the most common explanation they brought forward was that this was just soreness because I hadn't swum for a long time. I was swimming more like a beginner than an Olympic swimmer. Since I wasn't swimming vigorously, how could that cause soreness, let alone soreness that lasts for months? Others said I should hire a swimming instructor to make sure I was doing the strokes right. It's important to keep the core stable and only rotate the arms and shoulders.

I signed up for a private swimming lesson. I told my instructor I had back pain, so he gave me flippers to wear on my feet to make things easier. But instead of making it easier, my pain increased significantly. I didn't have the heart to tell him because I felt ashamed and didn't want to make him think that it was his fault that my pain had increased. He hadn't told me to do anything incorrectly—and I couldn't understand why this was happening.

I didn't return for any more classes but instead decided to teach myself how to swim. I already knew how to do some basics. In addition, I bought some excellent swimming DVDs and began to practice the drills for proper swimming. However, even after months of practice and improving my technique, the pain was no different.

Not wanting to quit on swimming, I bought a snorkel so I wouldn't have to rotate or twist my body. A body rotation is needed when taking a breath, so perhaps the rotation was impacting my spine and nerves. A snorkel allows you to breathe through a tube poking out of the water without turning your head to take a breath. But after swimming with the snorkel for a few days, it made no difference. The pain was still there, so apparently it wasn't caused by the rotation of my body.

After more research on swimming, I learned that backstroke is much better for the back than freestyle, the style I knew. Or I could try breaststroke, which is supposedly gentler on the back. I found out that backstroke uses almost exactly the same muscles as freestyle, so swimming backstroke made no sense. Nonetheless, I tried both backstroke and breaststroke, and they made my pain even worse.

I couldn't find anyone who was able to answer my swimming questions satisfactorily for me. I emailed my physical therapist, and she provided some standing aqua exercises I could practice in the pool without swimming. I tried them all, and they made no difference to my pain. I continued the physical therapy at home, and I continued to swim, hoping I would get strong enough to where my pain would go away. After all, I needed a strong core to support my spine, right?

I kept dreaming that after three months of swimming I would reach the requisite strength where the pain would go away. Maybe 20 lengths in the pool were not enough, it needed to be 30. Maybe even 40! Persistent, I pressed on and eventually made it to 40 lengths, which now—when I look back—is pretty good core fitness.

Between swimming and physical therapy, I was able to lead a diminished lifestyle where no one would know that I had pain, but I would simply avoid doing things that would cause it. On the outside I looked fine, but on the inside I was in constant pain or at the edge of pain. I've mentioned this a few times, and perhaps you feel the same.

Is your chronic pain an invisible illness?

One day I was in a bookstore, and as I pulled out a pen to write something, I dropped the pen on the floor. When I bent down to pick up the pen, I felt a searing pain shoot through my back and I fell to the floor. Oh no, not again! *What was the straw that broke my back this time?* People passing by simply thought I had got on the floor to pick up my pen. But I just lay there writhing in agony, unable to get up. Do your flare-ups return at the worst possible moments?

All those months of swimming had added up to *nothing* in that very moment I fell. The pain was as intense as ever, as if the swimming had never happened. I felt like I had just been betrayed by my most trusted friend. There are no words to describe the sadness and disappointment I felt in that moment, that the hopes raised by the last few months of swimming were completely dashed. Have you had moments like these?

Lying on the floor of the bookstore made me feel ashamed, so I grit my teeth through the pain, forced myself up, and returned home to rest.

Every two or three months something like this spasm would happen, and I would be back to square one. I would have to start my exercises from the beginning, and I would even have to start my swimming from the beginning, starting with two laps and then slowly increasing to four laps and gradually all the way back up to 40.

It was as if life were getting reset every two months, and I would start again from scratch. I felt like a windup toy that was being played around with. I kept asking myself what straw was breaking my back each time.

Despite the pain, I continued my swimming because it was the only exercise where I could exert myself and get an aerobic workout without immediately going into pain. I needed to keep my heart healthy. Perhaps you can relate to this too, because you too might be limited to only certain aerobic activities.

I would feel shame when people (especially women) asked me for help to lift things, move things, help with luggage, and so on. I would tell them I have back issues, and they would immediately tell me to be careful and would manage to do it by themselves. I remember visiting my mother, and my mother carried my suitcases for me. I felt so ashamed that my gray-haired mother had to carry my luggage. What kind of son am I?

> **Do you feel shame not being able to do some things for others?**

I skipped many social events because I knew I would be in pain sooner or later. Sometimes going to these events involved long drives, or playing physical games or dancing—neither of which I could participate in. I skipped any kind of physical events like camping, hiking, sailing, and canoeing, all activities within my reach but inaccessible to me. Friends would forget about my back pain and invite me, but when I would remind them, they would insist that it was not a strenuous activity, that even their 70-year-old dad could do it. Words like these hurt because I didn't feel understood.

Similarly, I would go to the grocery store and see much older people than me carrying heavy gallons of water with no pain. I would feel sad that, even though I look younger and stronger, a half gallon of water was about all I could manage. How I wished I could be normal!

I would eventually be normal—and you can too.

18
HOW IS YOUR POSTURE?

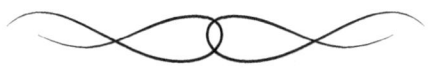

I had to find a solution to my pain. The instructions from my childhood about good posture came to me, and as I was researching online, I stumbled upon a book called *8 Steps to a Pain-Free Back*.

The author had suffered chronic pain after a pregnancy, and one day she made a connection between her pain and her posture. She began to observe the posture of people in developing countries compared to Western countries, and she noticed that people walk differently in developing countries versus those in the West.

Since I grew up in India and Africa, I was immediately able to connect to her message and notice that walking on hard pavement had changed the posture of Western people, while walking more often on grass and unpaved ground required a different kind of walking posture in developing countries. Even now, whenever I visit India, it takes me a week to get my "Indian legs." I keep tripping over things and stepping into potholes because the infrastructure isn't as well developed as in the United States.

I became convinced that this was the reason for my pain. If I could learn to walk differently, my pain would be gone. Having lived many years in the West, I had started to walk like Westerners. I was so excited about this process that I immediately signed up for her course and flew to Ann Arbor, Michigan, to take it.

She was a wonderful teacher, and during the weeklong class she showed us how we naturally walk and how in Western countries our walking has become more of a plodding along. She was definitely onto something here, because movie and stage actors spend years perfecting their walk and posture with coaches so that they look confident and attractive.

In this course I learned the eight steps for developing good posture and for walking correctly. During the class my pain lessened, and I started to have confidence that this was finally the solution to my pain. By the end of the week my pain was almost down to zero, and I was feeling incredibly hopeful.

Improving my posture through practicing this new method requires several months, and the teacher told me to take the time to perfect my posture and the way I walk.

I began diligently following these techniques and telling everyone I had finally discovered the source of back pain for myself and for everyone else who had back pain. I was sure I had found the answer. I was so confident I started giving out copies of her book to friends who were in pain.

For about two months my pain level was very low. I slowly began to increase my physical activities and do more and more things I wasn't able to do since the pain started. And the pain didn't return. One day I went to visit some of my friends who had an absolutely adorable two-year-old baby. Though I hadn't done this for a long time, I felt confident enough to pick up and hold the baby in my arms. As I held the child, I realized I felt no pain. I was excited; I had finally found a solution. I even told my friends that this posture class was working wonders and that I was able to hold their baby when I would have been afraid to do so in the recent past.

My becoming nearly pain-free in this situation was the result of the placebo effect. I will explain it in more detail in a later chapter. Have you ever found a method that seemed to work for a while?

It's interesting to note that in those moments when I felt I was completely healed, my pain would strike. Can you relate to this? As if on cue, the next day while I was sweeping my house, I felt a stabbing pain in my back, and once more my muscle spasmed. Not again! *What was the straw that broke my back this time?*

I fell to the floor crying because, once again, I had invested so much into this new technique, traveling to take the class, spending hours every day watching my posture, and yet after all that effort, here I was in pain again. It was as if I had never even taken the posture class—like the past few months had been a complete waste of time.

Frustrated and refusing to believe this wasn't working, and not willing to give up on this approach, I did a Skype session with the author of the book to try to understand what had happened.

> **Do you persist in continuing with methods that aren't working?**

The Straw That Broke the Camel's Back

She suggested that perhaps it was my psoas muscle that was injured and that I should rest for a while and then resume practicing the posture techniques. I was expecting a better explanation from her and was disappointed. That's what they all say, isn't it? Rest and then resume. This is such a common response, but no one explains why it isn't working.

However, my confidence in this new technique was now lost. How is it possible, when I have diligently learned a new way to walk, that my pain returns with the same intensity as before, as if it had never gone? I recall that this time, as I resumed my posture movements, the pain was especially intense, almost like mocking my attempt to try to escape it.

I fell into another depression, convinced I would never get out of this.

19
HOW DO YOU FEEL BEING ON MEDICATION?

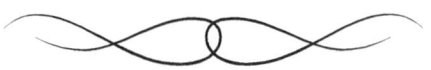

Living life at the edge of pain means not knowing what the next day will bring. Yet this was now my way of life, and I continued on. In 2016 my dad needed surgery, so I traveled to be with him. His surgery went well, and on the trip back home I was walking through the airport pulling my light rolling suitcase behind me.

Seeing someone running toward me, apparently late for a flight, I turned slightly to move out of the way and felt a twinge in my back. I prayed that this would not be the time I have a spasm; I needed to carry my luggage and sit during two connecting flights. I wouldn't be able to make it if I was in pain.

But as you may have experienced, the pain never comes at the most convenient moment, and within seconds the twinge turned into a full spasm. I sat down in excruciating pain and tears, wondering if I would be able to manage to make it home—with only eight hours to go. *What was the straw that broke my back this time?*

I never like taking medicine, but for moments like these I had packed some doses of diclofenac, which is a powerful pain killer that always works for me in the worst of pains. I took one pill and waited. And waited. But after half an hour it still wasn't working. I took a second dose, which isn't recommended so soon after the first, and waited. And waited. But this dose wasn't working either. My flight was boarding, and I managed to hobble into my seat and slump down while sliding my luggage under the seat because there was no way I could lift it to the overhead bin.

Eight hours later I arrived home, exhausted and in intense pain. The medicine hadn't worked, and I had been in level-9 pain the whole time. Again, recovery to my normal of 30 percent took another three weeks. This was the first time medicine had failed me. It was often my solution of last resort when the pain became unbearable. Have drugs ever failed you?

There is an opioid crisis happening in the world today. In 2018, in the United States alone, 130 people died every day from opioids because their pain was misdiagnosed.[15] Since the Covid-19 pandemic, this number has become much higher, more than 220 overdose deaths per day, for example, in May 2020.[16]

And the incidence of chronic pain around the world seems to be rising constantly.

What affect does medication have on you?

Drugs didn't work for my chronic pain. "They are just like applying lipstick," says Adam Heller, the founder of Zero Pain Now®. "They give temporary relief, covering up the pain. They only address the symptoms but not the cause of chronic pain."

And now, the one last resort I had—medication—had also stopped working. Could things get any worse? Oh yes, they could.

20
DO YOU FEEL YOU KNOW MORE THAN YOUR DOCTORS?

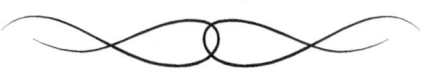

I was sharing my frustration with my father: "Dad, I don't understand when this pain comes and goes, and what I do to trigger it." He said, "Son, you are a scientific-minded person. Keep a record, take notes. Figure out what is going on. Research it. I know you can do it."

Encouraged by my dad, I continued on.

My engineering mind needed a solution, and I was determined to find the answer. There had to be a solution. Why can't my body heal itself? I read in anatomy books that if you break the largest bone in your body, the femur or thigh bone, it takes about six weeks to heal and then you're back to normal. Isn't that amazing?

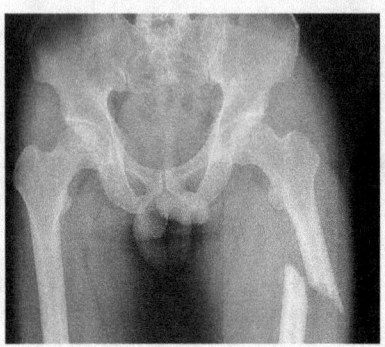

A fractured femur heals in about six weeks

And yet I was in pain for eight years. If it was a muscle that was injured, why didn't it heal? If it was a disc that was out of place or herniated, it should eventually shrink and its remnants get absorbed in the body. We have been around for millions of years, so how is it possible that such a debilitating condition can occur? Humans can be so physical—running, jumping, dancing—how can my spine be so fragile just by following a sedentary lifestyle or by sitting on a hard seat? If you've been told your pain is the result of an injury, why hasn't the injury healed?

What is more puzzling is why back pain wasn't that common in the distant past. Imagine running from a lion and suddenly you get intense back pain? You would definitely get killed and then your genes wouldn't pass on. So such a defect would have easily been filtered out by nature a long time ago. This doesn't appear to be a genetic issue as some people seem to believe.

Historical books rarely mention anything about chronic pain. Did any character in Shakespeare have chronic pain? Not that I can recall. Today one out of every two adults will experience back pain.[17] Chronic pain is a modern illness, and there are various explanations put forward for this. However, none of these withstand scrutiny when examined under a microscope. I have been eliminating these one by one for you as we go through this book. Let's keep eliminating the usual suspects.

But before that, a quick note on acute pain versus chronic pain. Acute pain is something that happens right after an injury such as a broken bone, a cut, a sprain. Acute pain usually heals within six weeks of an injury.

A few years ago my dad fell and broke his knee cap in two. Half of his knee was fractured and unusable. The fractured half of his knee cap was removed, and through the marvels of modern surgery, the surgeon tied the remaining *half of his knee cap* to his tendon using a wire. In seven weeks, the wire was removed, and he was back to having completely normal use of his leg, pain-free and jumping around like a little boy with only half a knee cap! I'm still amazed by the capability of modern medicine to perform miracles like this.

Modern medicine is amazing, and I have complete faith in it.

This statement might seem counter to this book, but you'll understand what I mean when you understand the solution. If it required a medical solution, researchers would have solved it well before now. When it comes to chronic pain, doctors cannot tell you with 100 percent certainty what the cause of the pain is or how it can be healed.

Chronic pain is usually defined as pain that lasts longer than three months. Personally, I would consider it to be pain that has lasted a year or longer. Sometimes pain just goes away in a matter of months and no explanation is required, but chronic pain keeps returning.

Why did my pain go away sometimes and then suddenly return when I sat on a chair? Sitting is such a harmless and benign activity. How can sitting cause pain? I would think that walking uses a lot more muscles, and yet I could walk for hours without increasing my pain. Walking was one of the few blessings I had, but somehow this made no sense if my pain was due to a structural issue.

It was time for me to turn to anatomy. No medical expert that I had seen until now, and I had seen many, had ever mentioned anything about my specific pain. All they did was show me pictures of the spine and how it moved, but nothing specific to what was happening to me. This should be a big clue in itself, that they might not even know what's going on. But I was about to discover this reason with more clarity as I dived into the details.

My posture teacher had mentioned that it was my psoas muscle that might be the origin of my pain, so I studied this muscle in detail. The psoas muscle is located in the lower lumbar region of the spine and extends through the pelvis to the femur. This muscle works by flexing the hip joint and lifting the upper leg toward the body.

I began to watch YouTube videos like a rabid medical student studying anatomy. Video after video after video. Not satisfied with the YouTube videos, I bought an excellent app called "Muscles and Kinesiology" by Visible Body, which included fantastic moving animations of all the muscles and bones in the body. You could remove layers of muscles until you could animate exactly the muscle and bone you were interested in, seeing the detailed origin and insertion points of how the muscles were connected to the tendons, which were connected to the bones.

While the app was fascinating, I soon explored the psoas and concluded that based on the location of my pain and the movements I was unable to do, it was not my psoas. For a few days I gave up, feeling deflated. Then I remembered from my physical therapy days that another muscle that's usually a culprit in back pain is the quadratus lumborum, often called the QL. The QL is the deepest abdominal muscle, though commonly referred to as a back muscle. I remember my physical therapist telling me that some of the exercises were for strengthening my QL. I started my app and studied the anatomy of the QL muscle, and with a startle I realized it was exactly the muscle that was spasming every time I was in pain.

Every kind of movement that the QL muscle facilitates, I was unable to do. Bending, twisting, carrying weights on only one side of the body. Yes, this was the muscle! I had diagnosed something no doctor or chiropractor had ever told me. I knew which muscle was spasming! I was close to a solution, and I would have something to teach them for a change.

What was even stranger was that it was only my left QL that would spasm. That was another thing I couldn't figure out. Why is the pain only on one side of the body?

My pain was off and on. It would start with a twinge at my left hip and then slowly move up to my lower back, at which point I would feel a great tightness in my left back. If I were then to do the wrong movement, the wrong lifting, or the wrong kind of sitting, the QL would immediately spasm and I would go into intense pain.

I wondered why the pain would move. I began to research how I could go about strengthening my QL. If you haven't noticed by now, I'm a research-aholic.

> **How many hundreds of hours have you spent researching your condition?**

I remembered that more than ten years ago I had injured my QL while carrying a suitcase when I was on a trip in Brazil. Perhaps this muscle had never properly healed and I needed to help it heal in some way. After all, injuries can lead to chronic pain, right?

I watched several YouTube videos on how to strengthen the QL muscle, and then began to do those exercises. I also purchased three tennis balls to lie on top of so I could do a deep massage of my QL muscle.

As I began to strengthen that muscle, I noticed that the pain decreased. I was feeling more and more confident that this time I really had found the solution. One of the exercises I used to do in physical therapy was the plank pose, where you lie on the floor face down, push up with your palms flat on the floor, and then hold the pose, keeping your body flat like a plank. My therapist had told me that if I could do the plank pose for one minute, I had excellent core strength. I also read that the plank pose is good for strengthening the QL.

So I slowly began to increase the time I was able to do the plank pose. I was at 30 seconds initially and slowly increased it to 45 seconds. While this sounds so easy to me today, when I was in pain, increasing 15 seconds felt equivalent to scaling Mount Everest!

I went to my chiropractor with this new information, and he told me that it was quite possible my QL was injured and that some scar tissue was left on the muscle. Since the QL is a deep muscle, it's not easy to heal the scar tissue. But he said there was a therapist in my area who had the technology to be able to heal the QL—the Graston Technique, which can be extremely painful but provide successful results.

Excited, I returned home and started to increase my QL strength even more. A few weeks later I was able to do the plank pose for an entire minute. I stood up jubilant and excited. Yes! *I know what muscle is hurt, and it's getting stronger.* My pain will soon be gone!

I'm sure you remember what happens the moment I feel happy, pain-free, and certain that I've found the solution. As before, this moment I was experiencing the pain-free placebo effect, which I will soon explain, and as if on cue, a few minutes after completing the one-minute plank pose, I felt a twinge in my lower back. And within seconds my QL spasmed and I collapsed on the floor writhing in pain. Not again! *What was the straw that broke my back this time?*

21
DID YOU GET A SECOND OPINION?

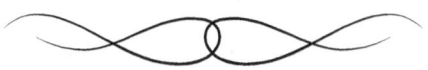

It was now seven years into my pain, and I had gotten used to living at 30 percent. I felt like a frog in pot of water that was getting hotter by the minute, and there was nothing I could do about it. I imagine you've learned to manage life with your chronic symptoms too. You've probably even forgotten what life was like when it didn't hurt. I had.

I was still convinced that my QL was the culprit. I decided that I was strengthening it too fast, that I wasn't giving it a chance for the scar tissue to heal between exercises. You may have noticed that sometimes it's not easy for me to let go of a belief—for example, my persistence with physical therapy, swimming, and the posture course. All these years the QL hadn't healed, so maybe the Graston Technique was needed.

Encouraged by the ideas of my chiropractor, I decided to get another MRI to clearly see if the muscle was damaged or if there were any newer structural defects in my spine before I went for the Graston Technique, which my insurance might not pay for because it was expensive.

This MRI involved many calls with my insurance company, doctors, and specialists within the medical system before I was able to get it approved. And after all that, I still had a large copay.

How much money have you spent treating your condition?

What was interesting was that the radiologist's findings concluded that nothing had changed in my spine in the last eight years. Seeing the second MRI was not as jolting as when I had seen the first. I was surprised and at the same time happy that at least nothing had become worse.

I took the second MRI to a new doctor, a world-renowned orthopedic surgeon for the back who had been practicing at the University of Miami for more than 40 years. Excited, I walked into his office and told him I knew exactly the source of my pain.

"Dr. Brown, I have figured out that the cause of my pain is my left QL muscle. Every movement I cannot do is linked to the QL muscle perfectly. My QL is broken."

"Mr. Singh, there is no such diagnosis. I've been doing this for 40 years, and I've never heard of a broken QL." He had a serious look on his face because, as I discovered later, muscles don't break. What I said hardly matched his medical knowledge. The conversation started to heat up.

I pulled out my MRI scans and showed them to him. "Look, this is where I'm getting the pain. All the movements are linked to the QL."

He looked at all my MRI photographs and said, "Mr. Singh, I cannot see any kind of damage to your quadratus lumborum from this MRI. Look at the QL on the other side. They are identical. Your QL is perfectly healthy. Your QL is not the problem." Apparently there was no scar tissue, so there would be no need for the Graston Technique. And today I can tell you that even if there was, scar tissue rarely results in chronic pain. If you've been told that scar tissue or an old injury is the cause of your chronic pain, it is false.

He turned to look at me and said, "Go home and stop doing everything you've been doing. Just go for 30-minute walks every day, that's all you need to do."

I was surprised. "How will I get my core strength?"

"That's easy, walking 30 minutes a day gives you all the core strength you need."

"Really?"

I left his office in confusion. Why hadn't anyone told me that before? Why was I doing months of physical therapy to strengthen my core? Why is there a whole industry around strengthening the core when all anyone has to do is walk? Is it possible that a strong core is useful only for good-looking abs but has nothing to do with back pain?

I had read many times that a simple walk can help heal your back pain. And hearing it from a renowned doctor who said my core would strengthen just by walking was good news.

Doctors have an amazing and vast knowledge when it comes to solving problems. I almost see them as engineers for the body. I found it hard to believe that doctors could not solve my problem. Why did every doctor I saw have a different opinion about the problem and a different suggestion for the solution?

I went home with mixed emotions. I had been convinced by my own research that my QL was the cause of my pain. But the doctor had looked at my MRI and said there was nothing he could see in the MRI that made him think my QL was anything but normal. My theory on my QL was now looking tenuous.

This was both good news and bad news. Good news because I didn't need a muscle transplant—yes, I had seriously Googled it to find out if a muscle transplant was possible! Bad news because it put me back at square one—with no answer to the cause of my pain. And on top of that he had told me to stop all my treatments and simply go for a 30-minute walk every day.

So I stopped doing my morning stretching and exercises and walked for 30 minutes every day. The good news was that nothing got worse; I stayed just the way I was. The bad news was that I wasn't getting any better. I was still living at the edge of a spasm, living at a physical ability of 30 percent, and if I were to do anything out of the ordinary, the odds were excellent that I would trigger a spasm.

In retrospect, I am sure with Dr. Brown's 40 years of experience, he must have realized that defects in the spine rarely cause pain, leading to his advice to stop everything and just walk.

22
WHAT ARE YOUR PAIN MANAGEMENT TOOLS?

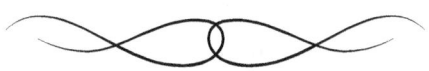

Over the years of managing my pain, I have amassed all kinds of devices to be able to do that. I imagine you have your set of tools for pain management as well. Here is a list of mine:

- TENS unit for high-voltage electrical stimulation of muscles
- Balance ball for exercise
- Massage devices
- Ice and heat packs
- Electric blanket
- Bone and muscle supplements
- McKenzie cushion
- Memory Foam car seat
- Three tennis balls
- Stretching strap

The Straw That Broke the Camel's Back

- Stretching rubber bands
- Back braces
- Shoe horn
- Medications
- Foot rest
- Special computer chair
- Under mattress support for my box spring
- A back cushion for sitting that I carried wherever I went

How many pain management tools do you have?

23
CHANGING THE LIGHT BULB

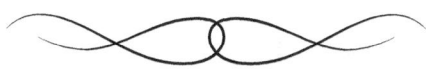

About two months passed and I had stopped my physical therapy and stretching. So far I had not had any spasms. I was feeling confident that maybe now I would heal. Perhaps just walking was the solution. Could it be as simple as this?

I was baking one day when my oven light blew out. I bought a replacement bulb and then had to open the oven door and lean toward the back of the oven to unscrew the old bulb. As I unscrewed the bulb and knelt on the floor, I was bending over with my head inside the oven. While I knew this was an awkward position, I felt confident that I was now healed. Yet once again I felt a twinge. I thought, No, I'm feeling fine, this isn't going to happen. But it did, and I felt as if a knife had slashed my back as my QL muscle spasmed.

I writhed on the floor in pain, and once again began to cry. I was sure, as I had many times before, that things were finally getting better. But clearly nothing had changed. I was still in the same condition, and there was no way to know when my muscle would spasm. *What was the straw that broke my back this time?*

Something I haven't mentioned before is that I keep a meticulous log of all my activities in an effort to trace back what might have caused my muscle to spasm. To find that straw that kept breaking my back. I wrote down that bending and twisting to change a light bulb causes me pain and to avoid that in the future.

Do you journal about your pain, trying to find a pattern?

I journaled because I noticed that my muscle would spasm for no reason, and so I needed to know what I had been doing yesterday to see if that caused the spasm. I still have this log and sometimes I look at it and laugh. It was my meticulous engineering mind keeping notes of all the clues. However, there was no clear correlation between what I did yesterday and when the pain came. No obvious straw that caused my spasm.

I looked at my log but couldn't find any activity that might have contributed to my spasm and pain. I was at the end of the line. My chronic back pain was the greatest mystery, and I knew I would not be able to solve it. I was getting close to the last straw.

24
HOW MANY SPECIALISTS HAVE YOU SEEN?

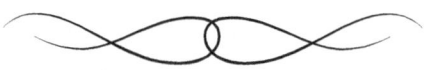

Throughout my years of pain, I saw several chiropractors. Some of my friends were treated by chiropractors regularly and suggested that I get another opinion from them. Instead of documenting my experience with each one, I've decided to summarize my experience with them in this chapter.

Something unusual would happen to me when I would visit a chiropractor. As I sat in the waiting room before I was called into the doctor's treatment room, my pain would diminish rapidly. I would sit there wondering, What am I doing at the chiropractor's office with hardly any pain?

I could never explain this phenomenon. It was almost as if I felt safe being in good hands, and my pain would go down. This again is the placebo effect, which I will explain soon.

Once I would meet the doctor, he would do the usual back cracking and neck cracking, and then he would ask me if I felt better. I would always say yes, and he would look pleased, but in all honesty I was already feeling better right before the visit.

And yes, you guessed it, once I left the chiropractor's office, the next day or even a few hours later, my pain would return.

Over the years that I saw chiropractors, here are some of the diagnoses and reasons they gave me for my pain:

The first one said I had an S-shaped spine and needed adjustments.

The second one said I had a pinched nerve and needed adjustments.

The third one said I needed preventive monthly alignments for the rest of my life, just like regular visits to the dentist.

The fourth one said I had a military neck and needed adjustments.

The fifth one said I needed to lie on the floor and rest my calves on my bed for half an hour every day.

The sixth one said I should never sleep on my stomach.

The seventh one told me I may have scar tissue and needed the Graston Technique.

What was surprising to me was that rarely would a doctor or chiropractor agree with each other. They all seemed to have a different opinion of what was wrong with me. Aren't these supposed to be the experts in their fields? And if the experts can't agree, isn't there something fundamentally flawed in their diagnosis?

Do you find that medical professionals are rarely in agreement about the solutions for your painful condition?

There didn't seem to be a common straw that would break my back. With our advancement of medicine and science, how can this be possible? How can we not pinpoint the cause of something so prevalent among billions of people? It's not like there is a shortage of numbers of people to study. This is not a rare disease.

This fact is itself a big clue to understanding the real cause of chronic pain—part of Sherlock's process of eliminating the impossible. If they can't find the straw in billions of us, maybe there is no straw to find.

"Things do not change; we change."

- Henry David Thoreau

25
THE LAST STRAW

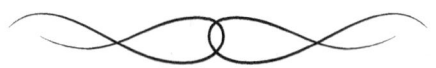

At this point I went into a depression. It had been eight years since my pain had begun, and nothing, absolutely nothing, that I tried had worked.

Attempting to get on with my life and out of depression, I signed up for a life coaching call, and the coach asked me, "What is the biggest obstacle in your life?"

"My back pain."

"Well, why haven't you done anything about it?"

"I have." I listed everything I had done.

"You have not done everything. You have found ways that didn't work. The only way you are going to solve this is to keep going. You need to get another opinion."

Angry at my coach for not letting me give up, I went to see a new doctor who came as an expert recommendation from a friend who is a doctor. The new doctor looked at all my previous results, and just like I expected, he prescribed more physical therapy. Reluctantly I went back to physical therapy, but this time much more knowledgeable about where my pain was and the exact muscle that spasmed.

This group of physical therapists was much better than my first, and they customized exercises based on where I was having my pain. They put me through a program that was more rigorous, having me lift heavier weights, work out my back on a back machine, bend side to side with a medicine ball, and undergo treatment with an ultrasound device to warm up my muscles before I began any workout.

At the end of the physical therapy, I would be massaged with a hot towel, and I would feel great, absolutely zero pain. This was amazing, I had never felt this good. Friends would joke that I was getting my insurance company to pay for a personal trainer. I didn't think this was very funny.

After about two months of therapy, I grew much stronger. But still, just like before, after my therapy session my pain would be almost gone, but the next day the pain would return. And when I went back to physical therapy, the pain would be gone again.

I asked my physical therapists why this was happening, why was it that when I came to physical therapy my pain would go away and then it would come back the next day. They would ask me what kinds of activities I was doing, and they noted there was nothing unusual in what I was doing. So they would shrug their shoulders and say they didn't really know.

Does your pain level increase and decrease without explanation?

Having physical therapy three times a week enabled me to max out the required weights for my back, my shoulders, and the bending exercises. Bending sideways had been a big fear for me, and I was happy now to be able to bend. However, because the pain would return the next day, over the weekends I would especially look forward to Mondays when I would be able to return to physical therapy.

After two months my physical therapy referral expired. I wanted to stay in therapy because the pain would still return the day after, but I needed to go back to my doctor to renew my referral.

This physical therapy had given me the best results. At least I was at zero pain after the ultrasound machine. So I decided to continue my physical therapy at home to see if I could maintain the partial success. The only thing I didn't have was the ultrasound machine. Each day I would spend at least two hours doing my stretches and exercises.

A few weeks later I attended a birthday party. When I left I walked out with a friend who was carrying a heavy bag of books. She asked me to help her carry them, and with my new sense of confidence, and feeling some shame when I thought about saying no, I agreed to carry her bag. I didn't know she was parked several blocks away, so I didn't expect to be walking so far. When we got to her car, I felt the pain starting to return.

Later that night I felt the twinge, and voila, I was back in bed. Back to square one. How often have you been back to square one? *What was the straw that broke my back this time?* I had had enough.

I went back to see my doctor to ask for a renewal of the therapy. He looked at the report from the physical therapists and said to me: "There is no point in renewing your physical therapy. I don't think there's anything we can do. You're stuck with this for the rest of your life."

> **Have you been told that your condition is lifelong?**

This conclusion was from a highly respected doctor. When I walked out of his office, I was sad, disappointed, angry, confused. I had also surrendered. I was at the last straw. I had given everything to fixing this problem, seen the best doctors and chiropractors and physical therapists. Maybe it was just time for me to accept that this is how life was going to be and make the best of it at 30 percent. At least I wouldn't have any more disappointments in trying something new.

"When I let go of what I am, I become what I may be."

- Lao Tzu

26
HAVE YOU SURRENDERED?

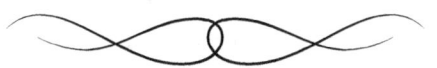

A few days later I was talking to one of my friends, telling him that sometimes in life there are no solutions. For an engineer like me this was a difficult concept to accept. I am a stubborn perfectionist and I like solutions. I do not like to surrender. But now I had surrendered. There was nothing more I could do that offered any promise of permanent success.

He listened to the story of my back pain, and he said he had recently heard of an audio book that, he was told, if you just listen to the book your pain goes away.

I laughed. "Really?"

This wasn't the first time a friend had told me of a new way to heal my pain. So I smiled to myself and thought, Great, here's another solution that is never going to work! I can't even be disappointed anymore.

So I agreed to listen to the book, even though in my mind I thought, I'm not going to bother but I don't want to disappoint him.

A few days later I was vacuuming my house. I was feeling good—in low pain—so I decided I might as well vacuum the whole place now because who knows when I will be feeling this good again.

> **Do you have bursts of energy in between your flare-ups?**

As I sat down to rest after I finished, I felt a little twinge in my lower back. No, please, not now. But yes, I had overdone the vacuuming, and within minutes my lower back spasmed. When my back spasms, my body goes out of shape, as if I were doing a hip bump with someone on the dance floor. I'm frozen into that awkward position. It sounds funny now, but it wasn't funny when I was in pain.

What was the straw that broke my back this time? Sad and frustrated, I lay down in bed and noticed on my phone that an email from my friend had arrived with a link to a copy of the audio book. I knew I would be resting for the next three days, and listening to an audio book while in bed was easy, so I decided to download and listen to this "magic" book.

What I heard changed my life, and it may change yours too.

"Everything should be made as simple as possible, but not simpler."

- Einstein

PART III
THE HEALING BEGINS

"Discovery consists of seeing what everybody has seen and thinking what nobody else has thought."

- Jonathan Swift

27
CAN WORDS HEAL YOU?

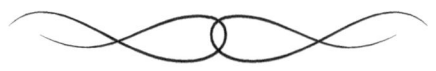

The author of the book was a rehabilitation physician who had done 30 years of research into chronic pain at the New York University medical center. He had suffered from chronic migraines and healed himself. Listening to his voice was comforting. He started explaining that for some people no amount of physical therapy or drugs or surgery helps. Yes, that's me!

He covered all the things people try—acupuncture, yoga, swimming, and so on—and these things seem to work for a while, but then the pain comes back. Yup, that's me!

He said chronic pain usually affects the deep body muscles of the back, shoulders, and buttocks. Yup, that's me too.

At this point I was listening very attentively because he was describing to a tee exactly what was happening to me. He said that if I have this condition it's very good news, because it means I can be healed. The pain is being caused by a mind-body connection.

Really? A mind-body connection? What's that? Isn't that woo-woo stuff?

With a gasp I realized that this was the exact book my doctor had suggested to me eight years ago when my pain had begun. And this was the exact book I had thrown into the trash because of a strange-looking amateurish drawing depicting an eye and a brain and thoughts.

I began to laugh and continued listening to the book. It was a different experience listening to it than reading it. And I was in a different place in my life now, having experienced all the ways that didn't work in trying to solve my pain. All the unidentifiable straws that I thought broke my back. About halfway through the book my pain decreased by half. When I finished listening to the book four hours later, I was feeling no pain.

I woke up the next morning, and there was still no pain. None at all.

What would it feel like for you to be completely pain-free?

I couldn't believe it. How could a simple book get rid of all my pain, let alone overnight? These were just words. My pain had never gone away overnight. Even if I felt low pain before going to bed, I would always feel pain in the morning. It took weeks to diminish the pain of a major spasm, and even then it was rarely at zero. There was something going on that I was about to discover that would change my life, and it may well change yours. It's simple and easy to understand.

Now, the important thing left for me was to *keep away my pain*, and in this regard, the book had some shortcomings. I will describe these shortcomings later, as well as the cause of pain. But before that, let's cover the placebo effect.

"The ultimate currency that rewards or punishes is often emotional."

- *Daniel Kahneman, Nobel Laureate, 2002*

28
THE PLACEBO AND NOCEBO EFFECTS

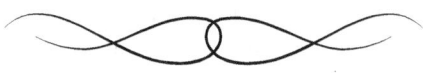

Now that my pain was gone, there was still a fear in me that listening to this book was a placebo, and that my pain would return. I had that happen so many times before. Yet something felt *right* about this solution.

Perhaps you've heard what a placebo is. The placebo effect is not well understood, but it is real and well documented in science. Sometimes the benefit of a drug is just the belief that the drug works and not the actual chemistry of the drug.

One example of the use of a placebo was during the Covid-19 vaccine clinical trials. When the vaccines for Covid-19 were being developed, the reason the release of the vaccines took so long was that they had to go through clinical trials where in half of the cases a real vaccine was used, and in the other half just an inert solution—a placebo—was injected into the trial volunteers. This was done to confirm that the vaccine chemistry was working and that the vaccine itself was not just a placebo. The vaccines available had much better results than the inert placebo.

The placebo effect occurs when a person strongly believes that something will work. In other words, the belief creates an absence of fear and a feeling of confidence. An absence of fear reduces stress in the body, and this allows the immune system to function at its best. Sometimes the immune system alone can rectify a problem without needing any drugs. This is the placebo effect. If a drug is no better than a placebo, it is rejected.

When it comes to chronic pain, the placebo effect also applies. When I went to see a chiropractor, I felt safe because I was with an expert who works with bones and nerves. There were usually impressive diagrams and models of the spine in the waiting room telling me this is an expert. And so my fear decreased and so did my pain.

The same thing appeared to be happening when I had physical therapy. Their job was to help me. They are the pain experts. *I felt safe with them.* And my fear would drop. And of course, physical therapy helps the *symptoms* of chronic pain, but not the *cause*, which was another reason I felt better during physical therapy but not after.

Does your pain level drop sometimes when you are feeling safe?

I've noticed on many occasions that when I'm feeling safe, my pain also decreases. And I've noticed the opposite: When I'm tense and under a lot of stress, my pain increases.

Every time I tried a new method, it seemed to work for the first few days—because I had a strong belief and hope that it would. But when my belief started to wear off, the pain would return. The physical therapy, swimming, stretching, medication, posture adjustments, acupuncture, yoga, and QL strengthening were all partial placebos and at the same time helping with the symptoms of chronic pain but not the cause. How were they helping with the symptoms? They were increasing blood flow to the area in pain. I will explain a little later why blood flow makes a difference.

The placebo effect explains why you find so many solutions for chronic pain when you Google for them. Some solutions do work simply because they create a placebo effect on the user, and this effect can last for some time—as long as you maintain a strong belief in the solution and keep your fear at bay and in turn your pain. And it's why you continue going for additional treatments—acupuncture, yoga, chiropractic adjustments, physical therapy—so you can reaffirm your belief in each treatment and keep the benefits of the placebo effect operating.

Another fascinating point is that if you do experience the placebo effect, it's encouraging news. It means that your back—or whatever area of your body has chronic pain—is fine and healable, and that you can get better using the solution described later in this book.

For me, it was momentous to know I had found the true cause of pain—the mind's effect on the body—and that the solution was not relying on a placebo.

The opposite of a placebo is a nocebo, referred to as the evil twin of the placebo. A nocebo has a detrimental effect on health produced by psychological factors such as negative beliefs or expectations relating to a treatment or prognosis. For example, people who strongly believe the Covid vaccine is harmful probably shouldn't get vaccinated. It could end up being a nocebo and cause increased stress and harm to their body and immune system.

I once saw a *Seinfeld* episode where someone died from licking envelopes when sealing the flaps because the glue was poisonous.[18] Since that day I no longer lick envelopes; I use water and my fingers to wet the envelope before sealing it. This is an example of a nocebo for me! Maybe it's silly, but I've programmed a nocebo in my mind.

All the notions from my past about touching my toes, keeping my back straight, bending at the knees when lifting, and keeping my core strong are all nocebos for me in the sense that I believe I will get back pain if I don't follow them.

My nocebo beliefs: Because I can't touch my toes, I'm inflexible, and therefore I will have back pain. My sedentary lifestyle leads to back pain. An injury to a muscle like my QL can lead to chronic back pain. Structural defects in the spine like the list of diagnoses from my MRI can lead to back pain.

Nocebos are all the beliefs that can lead to back pain (whether they are true or not), because they increase your stress and tension.

What are some nocebos you have about your chronic pain?

Take a few minutes right now and list your nocebos. Making this list will help you get better. If you know what your nocebos are, you can be more aware when you're acting under their influence and change your thoughts and actions.

After listening to the book, I was convinced that there is a mind-body connection to my pain and that if I can understand this mind-body connection, I will never be in pain again and will be freed from the whims of the placebo effect. I could clearly see a definite link between my stress and tension and my pain.

I hope you can relate to my journey, even though your pain may be different, your diagnosis may be different, and the solutions you tried may have been different. I suspect that your *emotional journey* was similar to mine. You've tried and tried and are still trying to end your pain. Stay with me, and soon you'll see how you can get better.

After we have tried everything, the only thing remaining must be the truth. You've tried enough, and it's not your fault. What I want to tell you is that this is exactly how we solve the mystery. You're probably stuck in the pain management cycle, and it's time to get out.

"I had therefore to remove knowledge, in order to make room for belief."

- Immanuel Kant

29
TRUSTING THE MIND-BODY CONNECTION

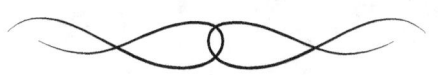

The audiobook I listened to, *Healing Back Pain: The Mind-Body Connection*, was written by Dr. John Sarno after he discovered the cause of many different types of chronic pain. He has been able to help tens of thousands of people to get better permanently. In 2012 he spoke to the US Congressional Senate Committee on Health to highlight the current chronic pain and opioid crises.

When I listened to his audiobook, I came to the understanding that everything I had tried was of a physical nature. I was trying to correct a structural defect in my body, to strengthen my muscles and core, to adjust my posture so that my body would function correctly without pain, and when necessary, to take drugs that would dull the edge of pain. These were all placebos or were temporarily increasing the blood flow to the part of my body that was in pain. Ultrasound was the best modality for me. When the ultrasound machine was applied to my back, I felt completely normal with zero pain. Now I realize that the ultrasound was a highly targeted device to increase blood flow in deep muscles. And of course, it worked; it is exactly the "indirect" solution required, which I will explain soon.

I also tried changing my diet and taking nutritional supplements, none of which made any improvement to my pain. I was not paying attention to any psychological processes in my mind. This is one of my favorite quotes from one of my favorite books:

> We are psychological beings, not logical beings.
> **Brad Blanton, Radical Honesty**

This explains why none of the physical treatments I had tried worked, because they addressed only the physical or structural issues of my body. I had been continually asking all the doctors and specialists I had been seeing which muscle this exercise was strengthening, what nerve controlled this muscle, which bone connected to this muscle. I couldn't help but notice that I didn't get any answers. I didn't get any congratulations about figuring out that it was my QL that was spasming. I didn't get an explanation why the pain was on the left side of my back and not on the right. I didn't get an explanation about why when I sat down I had pain, but when I walked my pain would decrease. I didn't get an explanation why sometimes my pain would go away and just randomly come back. I didn't get an explanation why sometimes physical therapy would take away my pain and sometimes it would make my pain worse.

At some point I think I even stopped asking the questions because I started to believe my questions were dumb when I noticed the faces of my therapists scrunch up. But the honest truth is, the answer wasn't there, the answer isn't a structural issue. It was not their fault that they didn't know, and now I understand that they don't know that they don't know.

In the morning after listening to the audiobook, I woke up pain-free because I realized that if my pain was a structural issue, my body would have healed itself. Structure was not the straw that broke the camel's back. I felt safe waking up in the morning because I became convinced my back was fine. And you too will discover your body is fine.

I imagine you're going through experiences with doctors similar to mine. You probably have short meetings with them, after which they want to send you away, give you drugs, prescribe physical therapy, or give you some other standard response. When you ask them questions, they simply repeat one thing over and over again, until you feel stupid that you're even asking. The truth is they don't know the answer, even though they do care and want to help.

I also realized why I had thrown this book into the trash eight years earlier. I wasn't ready to hear the answers. From my childhood I have been conditioned to believe that back pain is a structural issue. Because I couldn't touch my toes, I was going to have back pain; because I was slumping in my chair, I was going to have back pain; because I was leading a sedentary lifestyle, I was going to have back pain; because my car seat was hard, I was going to have back pain; because my dad had a slipped disc, I was going to have back pain—and so on.

Messages and beliefs I had adopted from the world around me had conditioned me to believe that my pain was a physical issue. However, all the experts I saw were not paying attention to anything specific to my pain. They were simply pushing me into a pain management cycle. It was a machine that addressed symptoms but not the cause. Each solution should be very specific to the problem, if the problem is truly physical. The book pointed out a list of glaring statistics that are completely ignored even though they are published in the most famous of medical journals. I've listed a few of these throughout this book, which clearly indicate that the problem is not conclusively structural.

I have to be honest that my first doctor was the best *and I didn't understand him.* He told me that some people have the structural defects and have pain, and some people have the same structural defects and have no pain. And he had recommended the book that I promptly ordered and then later trashed.

Medicine is filled with supporting facts that many people have structural defects and have no pain. Here are a few facts I will list again for you, plus some new ones:

1. A study published in *The New England Journal of Medicine* shows that MRIs on 98 people with *no pain* included 66 percent with bulging discs or herniated discs.

2. A study in the *Journal of Pain Research* indicates that back surgery success is at 35 percent. Why would this number be so low if back pain was a structural issue?

3. A study published in *The New England Journal of Medicine* shows that people with osteoarthritis improved equally well regardless of whether they received a genuine surgical procedure for a knee or a fake one.[19]

4. The prevalence of low back pain by the age of 20 was up 80 percent in 2011.

5. The number of people in chronic pain is increasing and currently estimated at 1.5 billion.

6. Opioid death rates are increasing because pain medication is being incorrectly prescribed. Big Pharma companies have been sued for $26 billion in lawsuits just like the tobacco industry was sued in the 1990s.[20]

7. The annual cost of chronic pain is at $600 billion, which is more than heart disease, diabetes, and cancer combined.[21]

8. A study by neurosurgeon Dr. H. L. Rosomoff shows that less than 3 percent of the cases of back pain are related to a structural issue that requires surgery.[22]

9. A pain medicine doctor, L. Johnson, said, "Just about any approach is better than having surgery because all the studies have shown that if you take a surgical population and nonsurgical population they all seem to do the same in 5 years."[23]

These facts corroborate the success rate at Zero Pain Now®, where we are able to help more than 90% of people with chronic pain get permanently better without drugs, surgery, or physical therapy.

I will now get into what the mind-body connection really means, and how simple it is, so you can understand it and get better.

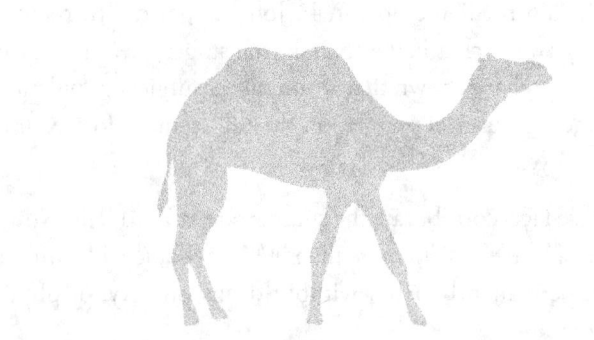

"It is what we already know that often prevents us from learning."
- *Claude Bernard*

30
A TRAFFIC SIGNALING ANALOGY

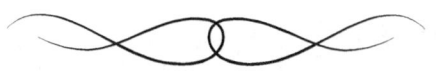

A communications system is made of two parts: a traffic network and a signaling network. It's like an information highway. For comparison purposes, imagine the road networks that we drive on. It's the same concept. There are the roads, and there are the traffic lights to control the traffic on the roads. These are separate networks.

In the same way, our body also has a musculoskeletal system—the roads—and a nervous system—the traffic signals. These are separate systems.

The mind-body connection is at work when the mind sends a signal through the nerves to a part of the body.

The medical community focuses on two things for chronic pain, the body and the nerves:

1. They look for a flaw or injury in the body—a muscle, tendon, bone, or organ.

2. They look for a blockage in the nerves, like a pinch.

This makes a lot of sense. These are the usual suspects. And there can be good reasons for these issues, like cancer or organic disease. In these cases, *medicine can solve it*.

However, when it comes to chronic pain, medicine has examined these cases with a microscope and has not found a solution. Medicine has only found a way to treat the symptoms. Given how predominant chronic pain is in our lives, what might surprise you is how little training doctors receive for pain medicine while they are in medical school.[24]

> Doctors in the US spend 11 hours learning about pain medicine in medical school.
> **Pain and Therapy Journal**

And so, like Sherlock Holmes, we must eliminate the impossible, and the only thing left is the truth. What is the only thing left? Medicine fails to investigate one important part of the picture: the central controller, our mind. To complete the traffic signaling analogy, every major city has a traffic control center where they can change the timings of the traffic lights. You have probably seen this control center in movies when the bank robbers take control of the traffic lights and create havoc in the city to make sure their getaway car gets all the green lights.

In our body this central controller is the mind. It turns out the real problem is that the wrong *signal* is being sent to the body from the mind. The good news is that the body and the nervous system are *fine* and healthy. Even better news is that the mind is *fine* too. It just needs to be made aware that it's sending the wrong signal.

Imagine a lightning strike or a power outage at a traffic light. Chaos ensues on the streets, right? There is a traffic pileup and congestion. But pretty soon people adapt and traffic continues to flow slowly. A policeman comes and guides the traffic with his hand signals. Then the utility company comes out and fixes the light. Traffic resumes, and everything is back to normal. And stays normal. This is how the body can heal itself. This is what happens when there is a pain from an acute injury; for example, my dad breaking his knee cap, or any kind of serious accident.

But what if the traffic light was sent the wrong message from the central controller? No amount of fixing the traffic lights or patching the roads would relieve the chaos. Because the traffic light and the roads are fine. The message from the central controller is wrong. This wrong message can develop after an acute injury has physically healed. The mind keeps sending that pain signal because that signal is believable: "After all, I had a sports injury there, didn't I? So the pain makes sense!" The mind is aware of all your nocebos and can direct the signal to those parts of the body.

And the mind can send the wrong message to different parts of the body. This is why it's common for the pain to move around. For me, it would start at the hips, move into my lower back, and then finally spasm my QL. For people with CRPS and fibromyalgia, the pain is in many places at once. This is why so many different chronic pain diagnoses can be healed with the same correction to the message.

Medicine addresses the symptoms of chronic pain but not the cause. Because the symptoms will always be there to some degree, medicine focuses on pain management. The result? A $600 billion chronic pain industry. The opioid crisis.

The regular visits to acupuncturists, chiropractors, and all the other pain management treatments many of us in chronic pain are getting. I was spending hours daily managing my pain.

> **How much time do you spend daily managing yours?**

We are fixing the roads and traffic signals, which seems to be the logical thing to do. But it turns out they're fine. Trying to fix the roads and traffic signals is a never-ending task because they're not the problem. The problem is that the message being sent is wrong. Addressing the cause (the message) fixes all the symptoms. This is called pain banishment—no monthly visits, just a permanent solution once you understand why the wrong signal is being sent.

This is a partial explanation of the mind-body connection. The brain sends an incorrect message to the body, and the result of this message causes pain. And it's very easy to correct this signal. Once the message is corrected, the pain vanishes.

The solution is similar in a communications system. In my more than twenty years of working in telecom, the majority of the problems I encountered were the messages themselves, not the signaling path the messages traversed or the hardware of the network. A breakdown of the hardware or the fiber optic cable was easy to diagnose and correct. We could fix a communications system in minutes once the breakdown was identified. You find the part that is broken, and repair it or replace it. Simple. Problem solved.

However, an incorrect message resulted in incorrect actions, unusual erratic behavior, problems that appeared sometimes and then disappeared. Occasionally this could take weeks and months to troubleshoot and solve. The physical structure of the system was fine; it was just doing what the messages told it to do. The problem was that the messages were wrong from the central controller. And these were the trickiest issues to solve.

But once you understand the mind-body connection, the solution—changing the message—is much easier than fixing a communications signal.

> "Where so many hours have been spent in convincing myself that I am right, is there not some reason to fear I may be wrong?"
> - *Jane Austen*

31
THE MISTAKES I MADE

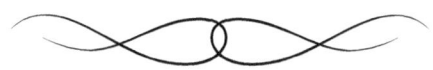

Let's recap the mystery again from the beginning and see how the clues misled me:

Nocebos that resulted in a belief that I would get back pain:

1. I was unable to touch my toes.

2. I didn't sit up straight.

3. My dad had a slipped disc.

4. I didn't bend my knees when lifting.

5. I saw messages in the media conveying that the back is fragile, e.g., Andre Agassi, NFL players.

6. I bought a new car with tight bucket seats.

7. I began working from home, leading a sedentary lifestyle.

Results of my nocebos:

1. I started to get back pain.

2. I saw a doctor, and he found defects in my spine and recommended injections, physical therapy, and a book on the mind-body connection.

3. I went to physical therapy and later practiced the recommended exercises on my own.
4. I attended a yoga class.
5. I practiced the McKenzie Method.
6. I went to an acupuncturist.
7. I started swimming.
8. I attended a posture course.
9. I took medication.
10. I used heat and ice and a TENS device for my pain.
11. I studied anatomy and strengthened my QL.
12. I had a second MRI.
13. I was back in physical therapy, and the ultrasound helped temporarily.
14. My doctor told me I had my condition for life.

The methods included in this list were all pain management approaches to increase blood flow, which gave me temporary relief. (I will soon explain why blood flow relieves pain.) And many of these were initially placebos because, starting them, I would be excited that I might finally get better.

Below are facts that cast doubt on contemporary solutions for chronic pain:

1. Younger people are in pain more than ever.
2. Back surgery success rates are dismal, yet people still do them because they are in so much pain.

3. Most knee surgeries have been shown to be a placebo.

4. More and more people are experiencing chronic pain.

5. Thousands are getting permanently better by using the mind-body connection solutions.

6. More doctors are referring chronic pain patients to a mind-body process to get better.

These clues to the mystery are obvious to me now. Some of these structural solutions might be the clues you are chasing. You may have different placebos and nocebos, but your experiences are likely similar to mine. Some things work sometimes, some things don't work, and you have your own triggers that set off your pain. For me, the things that triggered my pain were sitting, twisting, lifting, running, dancing, and bending. If you can relate to this, there is an excellent chance you can get better.

All the false clues I had investigated finally led me to the mind-body connection. What is the mind-body connection, and what does blood flow have to do with it? What's the incorrect message from the mind that causes pain? Let's move on to the details of the *cause* now.

"There is nothing new except what has been forgotten."
- *Rose Bertin to Marie Antoinette*

32
THE CAUSE

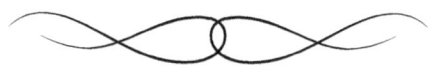

Dr. John Sarno had found the cause of chronic pain: the mind-body connection. But what does this really mean? If you've been reading this book from the beginning, this will be easy to understand.

Let me first illustrate with an example. Remember a time when you were afraid. I imagine that the blood rushed out of your face. Maybe you were even trembling.

This is what's happening with chronic pain. Stress and tension lead to certain emotions with negative effects on the body. These emotions lead to a reduction in blood supply. Reduction in the blood supply leads to a reduction in oxygen in some part of your body. And a reduction in oxygen leads to pain, burning, tingling, numbness, or weakness in that body part. Swedish researchers and many others have documented a reduction in oxygen in the tissues of back pain patients. In medical language this reduction of blood flow is called ischemia.

> Oxygen deprivation was noticed in the muscles of back pain patients.
> **Fassbender and Wegner**

Similar oxygen deprivation was reported in studies with patients diagnosed with fibromyalgia.[25] Such studies showing oxygen deprivation at sites of chronic pain have been well documented in medical literature. This is a mild oxygen deprivation, about 3–5 percent, which can result in excruciating pain, even though it doesn't harm the body. And the pain is very real and not in your head!

Dr. Sarno noticed that people who were suffering from chronic pain were not aware of the emotions causing the reduction in blood flow. He therefore called these *repressed emotions*. Another way to look at repressed emotions is to say that the mind is *disconnected* from certain emotions.

That's it. It's as simple as that. The disconnection causes the brain to send an incorrect message, which reduces blood flow. The reduction of blood flow causes numerous manifestations of pain experienced in the body of chronic pain sufferers. The symptoms of these include some or all of the following: *pain, burning, tingling, numbness, and weakness.* In Zero Pain Now® terminology this is called a *psycho-physical reaction*. The reaction originates in the mind and triggers an event in the body.

This explains why physical therapy, swimming, ultrasound, and heat pads were all working for me. These increase blood flow, which in turn increases oxygen to the body part and then reduces the pain. Imagine the heat and exercise and movement as the policeman helping the traffic to flow at the broken traffic light, and imagine that the traffic represents the blood flow. The moment my therapy session with these modalities ended, my pain would return. And when I first tried these modalities, I would have great success due to the placebo effect as well as the increased blood flow. Once the placebo effect wore off, I would only have momentary success with the modality from the temporarily increased blood flow and oxygen, and then the pain would return once I stopped the therapy.

Dr. Sarno also found that the solution to healing from chronic pain was two simple steps.

Step one: The mind has to be convinced that the pain is not structural. In other words, the body is fine, the nerves are fine, the mind is fine.

Step two: Become consciously aware of the repressed emotions, and the reduction of blood flow and oxygen will no longer occur. Once the patient is aware of the emotions, the emotions pass through and no longer cause any physiological changes and the related pain. The cause is gone and so is the pain.

By listening to his book, I had accomplished step one of the process. I was already feeling better. I was confident about having found the solution, and I had lost the fear of having a fragile spine. I didn't need a spine transplant.

For those of you reading who have a structural diagnosis, embracing step one is vital, though it may not be easy to believe. My friend Gayle slipped down several flights of stairs after a water main accident flooded her apartment. She fractured her spine in 63 places. Her doctors told her she would be in a wheelchair for the rest of her life and might even die within six years. After recovering in due time, she's walking normally and living well past her predicted timeline. Our bodies, combined with modern medicine, are incredible healing machines.

For those of you reading who do not have a structural diagnosis, good news, you only have to cover step two!

As for me, I am an engineer, and by my nature I'm not an emotionally aware person, so I knew that step two might take me a little more time. What does it mean to be connected to my emotions? I have an introverted personality. Does it mean I have to be outgoing and extroverted? Does it mean I have to share how I'm feeling with other people? Does it mean I have to change who I am? I had all these questions in my mind.

I felt connected to my emotions now that I was pain-free after listening to Dr. Sarno's audiobook. How and why was I disconnected from my emotions in the first place? And what if I begin to disconnect from my emotions again? I never want to be in pain again!

> **I decided I would learn to connect to all my emotions, *whatever* it took.**

What I learned is that I didn't have to be outgoing, extroverted, or share my feelings with anyone, or even change who I was. More good news.

Let's continue to Step 2 of this solution so you can understand it in more detail.

"It is always the simple that produces the marvelous."

- Amelia Barr

33
UNDERSTANDING STEP 2

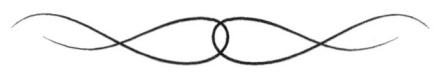

One of the shortcomings of Dr. Sarno's program is that for Step 2 he required people to see a psychotherapist because he didn't have a simple process to free up repressed emotions. Seeing a psychotherapist is expensive and also means several months of often unnecessary therapy. I didn't want to go through months of therapy. I was now pain-free and wanted to stay pain-free. So I began to search for methods to follow Step 2, to become consciously aware of my emotions.

That's when I discovered a program called Zero Pain Now®. The creator of Zero Pain Now®, Adam Heller, had extensively studied neuroscience and pain for more than 20 years, including Dr. Sarno's process. He discovered a simple method that can be practiced by anyone to reconnect to their emotions without psychotherapy.

Adam has already helped over 4,000 people become permanently pain-free. He did a proof-of-concept study with a major medical clinic in the United States using his process of connecting to emotions. In this pilot 100 percent of the patients presented to him were pain-free within 28 days. His process was so simple that by day six, 85 percent of his clients were pain-free. I will describe this process later in more detail.

Imagine that you have been suffering for years and years and have come across this program where between 6 and 28 days you can become pain-free and be able to get back to doing everything you have always dreamed of doing. You just have to change the signal from the mind and build that change into a habit.

Hard to imagine, right? I was definitely skeptical. But it's because I had spent years trying to fix the wrong thing. Once you find the cause, the fix is immediate, the traffic light starts to function correctly. It really is possible to quickly stop pain once you address the cause.

So I signed up for Adam Heller's program, and within days of starting, I too had excellent results. My pain didn't return, and I began to increase my physical activity. The program was easy to do right at home and followed a prescribed and proven process. By following Adam's program, I have now been pain-free for five years. Not a single spasm, which was happening almost every two months before this! I now have the tools to keep myself pain-free—tools to make me aware that my mind is sending the wrong signals and that there is no real injury to cure. I am fine.

Dr. Sarno was the groundbreaker for discovering this solution and may be compared to the Wright brothers when they made the discovery of flight with a simple wooden propeller aircraft. Adam has advanced this discovery. Adam's Zero Pain Now® program is like the invention of the jet aircraft, streamlining the original discovery of permanent pain relief, making it targeted, fast, and simple.

What was my emotional disconnection that started my pain? It will help you to understand what happened to me.

"There is nothing either good or bad, but thinking makes it so."
- *William Shakespeare*

34
THE STRAW THAT BROKE MY BACK

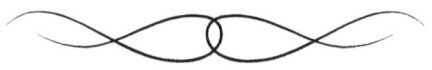

Let's complete the mystery of what was the cause of my pain, what was the straw that broke my back.

Remember that chronic pain is caused by a disconnection from certain emotions. More specifically, chronic pain is caused by a disconnection from certain emotions *that usually conflict with your self-image*. Because of this, no psychotherapy is required. A simple process connects you back to your emotions, and a 28-day period of forming the habit to make this connection becomes as automatic as walking. Or dancing—which you might spontaneously feel like doing once you're pain-free.

I will tell you the straw that broke my back. Just like a good mystery, the clues to the crime were right in the beginning. It is important that you read my story at the beginning of this book so you can appreciate the simplicity of the clue. If you remember, my pain began after my employer of 15 years filed for Chapter 11 bankruptcy. I started working from home with long hours of work, a sedentary lifestyle, and a lot of stress.

When a company files for Chapter 11 bankruptcy, its stock becomes worthless. I didn't know that at the time. Management had told me that our company was financially stable and that we would never file for Chapter 11. They specifically told all the employees that we had $4 billion in cash to protect us.

On the day that my employer filed for bankruptcy, I also learned that I had lost almost all my retirement savings, which were invested in the company's stock. There is no grace period for this filing. No 24-hour notice. No warning. No internal memo. Our management had denied we were in financial trouble. I had invested a substantial amount of money in my company's stock over the previous 15 years for my retirement. It was more than a hundred years old with a large customer base and an established reputation. No one could have imagined it would be mismanaged into bankruptcy. Worse, after declaring bankruptcy, our management told us not to worry, that we would come out of bankruptcy so there was still nothing to worry about! But it didn't bounce back. The show was over. It no longer exists today.

How do you deal with a significant event in your life?

When I look back at that day, I remember I went numb, disconnected from any emotions. What could I do? Absolutely nothing. There is no protection for money in the stock market, even if it is retirement savings. There was no one I could write to. There was nowhere I could file a complaint. There really was nothing I could do. In fact, even today I can do nothing. My emotions were so repressed I couldn't even identify them at the time. How would that make you feel, to lose most your life savings of 15 years in one day? The emotions that were bubbling underneath my numbness were fear, shame, sadness, anger, and rage—and I wasn't aware of them.

Hopefully you wouldn't respond the way I did. Imagine a movie scene where the hero loses his life savings. He'd probably smash up the place and yell and scream at his boss. That's why actors get paid a lot of money. Not me. I played it cool. By the way, I'm not saying you have to smash up the place. That's done in a movie so the audience can understand how the actor feels. All I had to do was allow myself to feel those emotions. Instead, I numbed myself to them.

Since there was nothing I could do, I didn't want to feel my emotions because I didn't know what would happen if I did, *not realizing what would happen if I didn't*. And that's exactly what causes chronic pain—a disconnection from certain emotions that you really don't want to feel because you don't know what would happen to you if you did, usually resulting from an event that you can do nothing about. The emotions conflict with your self-image of being someone who's in control of their emotions and their life.

Most people in chronic pain are already quite good at disconnecting from emotions just based on their personality type (more on this later). When a significant emotional event happens to them, it solidifies this behavior, cements it in.

Then, once you start disconnecting from some of your emotions, the problem starts compounding. Not only does that disconnection become a habit, but you start noticing that the pain comes when you do certain activities. You associate the pain with an activity instead of associating it with your emotions. For example, for me the pain would come when I would drive my car sitting on a hard seat. So my mind makes the connection that the seat is what is causing the pain. This trains my mind to create neural connections that trigger my pain.

All the time I was driving my new car, I was going through the stress and tension of the events happening at work, trying to keep from getting laid off, and wondering what my future was going to be now that I had lost my life savings. Wondering why the company leadership had not warned me what to prepare for. Not only was it the only company I had ever worked for, it had almost become my family because I had been there so long and become close to many of my fellow employees. It felt like a family betrayal.

I associated all the emotions arising from the stress and tension of the situation to the stiffness of my car seat and my sedentary lifestyle, sitting for hours at home slumped over my computer. If you've heard of Pavlov's dogs, who would drool when he rang a bell signaling that food was coming,[26] then this is exactly what started happening with me. And over the years, I made more and more connections until many simple things started triggering the pain: sitting on chairs, sitting in movie theaters, sitting on barstools, or bending or twisting or dancing or vacuuming or just changing a simple light bulb. Reflect a moment on this question:

What triggers your pain?

The problem compounds quickly to the point where the mind is convinced that something is wrong physically or structurally in the body because certain physical activities seem to cause the pain—along with all the related nocebos. In reality it's simply a disconnection from an emotion that has triggered this whole series of events—an incorrect message sent by the brain to the body. Different people can have different triggers for the same pain. Some people get pain in the morning, some in the evening, some while running, some while sleeping, and I'm sure you have your own list of triggers for your pain. I've even heard of a person who gets back pain when it starts snowing. Everyone has their own straws that they think are the ones that broke their back.

The collapse of my company and all my corresponding repressed emotions were the straw that broke my back. Ironically, the rest of the evidence—structural defects, weak core, flexibility, sedentary lifestyle, injury, etc.—were merely *diversions*, a false trail that led me to eight years of more pain. Understanding this diversion is your path to healing, knowing that you can get better.

"You can outdistance that which is running after you, but not what is running inside you."

- *Rwandan proverb*

35
DIVERSION PAIN SYNDROME

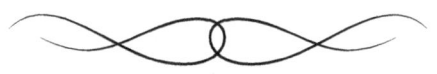

Adam Heller has named this condition of disconnecting from emotions as the Diversion Pain Syndrome (DPS). The definition of DPS is:

> **To divert your attention from an unbearable emotion to something physical like pain.**

This is a revealing definition that is worth rereading several times. Let's relate it to my example. I lost 15 years of savings in one moment. I went numb. Apparently I didn't want to feel my emotions. They were too unbearable. These emotions—I now know—were fear, sadness, shame, anger, and rage—and probably a few more. My hard-earned money was "stolen" from me. I was misled by my company leaders who had mishandled the company finances, declared Chapter 11, received golden parachutes, and got away scot-free.

I don't know what I might've done if I had allowed myself to feel these emotions, so I buried them so deep I wasn't even aware of what the emotions were. And because I repressed them, my mind diverted my attention from these emotions "to something physical like pain." Today I know that nothing will happen if I allow myself to feel the emotions; they are just emotions and they will simply flow through me.

As already mentioned, I'm a perfectionist and not an emotional person to begin with, so my personality also compounds this condition. I had probably been repressing many other emotions, without knowing it, earlier in my life. I will talk about personalities in the next chapter.

Have you noticed a link between stress and tension and your pain?

"What was the straw that broke my back this time?" Every time I wrote this line in my pain journal, I was experiencing stress and tension in my life, which was triggering my pain. I wasn't aware of the corresponding emotions, so I wasn't even noting them down.

The healing process begins with connecting to all your emotions, the ones you feel and especially the ones you are repressing and not only don't know about, but don't want to know about. It's common *not* to feel these emotions because they conflict with your self-image, thus making them unbearable. So people starting this healing program may not immediately know the emotions they are repressing.

Have you ever driven home on autopilot without realizing how you got there? Sometimes this happens to me. Or having misplaced something, when you find it, having no idea when you put it there? Numerous scientific research has shown that more than 95% of our brain activity is unconscious.[27] This is similar to not being aware of the emotion that is being repressed. Sometimes things are *out of our awareness* until we consciously put our awareness onto them.

Please stop reading now and take about five minutes to ponder the following question. Be honest. Journal freely for a few minutes if you need do.

What was going on in your life when your pain began?

Part of the process of the Zero Pain Now® program is journaling to catalog all your emotions and bring them to the forefront so you are aware of them and then build a habit of being connected to all of them. The solution is really that simple. The secret to success is just to allow this process to work for you. The Zero Pain Now® program has a 95 percent success rate in helping clients get pain-free, and more important, to stay pain-free.

Zero Pain Now® is classified as a biopsychosocial program, which means it leads with the premise that evaluating a person's medical condition does not simply focus on biological factors, but also psychological and social factors.[28] The US Department of Health and Human Services (HHS) report on pain management best practices recommends "Emotional Awareness and Expression" programs as an alternative to opioids for chronic pain.

Healing is not complete until the four goals of Zero Pain Now® have been met:

- Little or no pain
- Back to physical ability
- No more drugs or tools
- No more fear

As you can see, the criteria for success is specific and strict to ensure that the pain reduction is not a placebo, and that the healing is permanent and you are pain-free for the rest of your life.

Once my pain went away, I started increasing all my physical activities. I can now easily swim 40 lengths of the pool and not even be out of breath. I give my friends piggyback rides just because I can. I can run and play any sport I enjoy. I started taking dancing classes because I am no longer in pain when I twist and turn. Dancing is freedom for me. It tells me I am fine.

I no longer spend hours every day in pain management: stretching, exercising, or taking any kind of medication. I haven't stretched for years. I'm sure stretching is great for flexibility, but I found out the hard way that it makes no difference to chronic pain.

I am completely pain-free, and more important, I'm constantly aware of my emotions, which gives me far more benefits than just being pain-free. I can sleep better and even my seasonal allergies have disappeared. I am more assertive and able to draw clear boundaries in my interactions with other people.

Now that you understand the cause, let's talk about some more factors that can make you susceptible to disconnecting from certain emotions.

"The person most in control is the person who can give up control."

- Fritz Perls, founder of Gestalt therapy

36
ARE YOU A PERFECTIONIST?

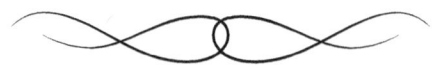

This chapter is about how our personalities can contribute to that disconnection, leading to chronic pain. This chapter might surprise you, because I'm going to tell you something that is counter to everything you may have learned. If you are in pain, you need to stop being *only* positive. Let me exemplify what I mean.

I'm a very positive person. Who would disagree with positivity? Let's look at my positive behavior from real-life examples.

Example 1: Oh no, my life savings are worth almost zero and my company is bankrupt!

Oh, that's OK, I'm still young and I can recover from this. I can learn from my mistakes. I'm still OK and I still have a job. Yay!

Example 2: Oh no, my girlfriend just ghosted me. She moved out of my apartment without even saying good-bye!

Oh, that's OK. The relationship wasn't going that well anyway. It's better we are apart and at least we didn't have an angry confrontation and a dramatic breakup. I'm sure I'll find someone right for me and so will she.

Can you relate to such positivity for situations in your life?

As human beings we are multidimensional; we have a full range of emotions. By being "positive only," I was missing out on allowing myself to experience emotions I didn't want to feel. These emotions are usually called negative emotions because there's a tendency to avoid them.

Below is one of my favorite quotes, from social scientist Brené Brown's book *The Gifts of Imperfection*. Allowing yourself to feel all your emotions makes life fuller and brighter.

> "We cannot selectively numb emotions. When we numb the painful emotions, we also numb the positive emotions."
> **Brené Brown, The Gifts of Imperfection**

Let's imagine emotions as colors. Suppose I like the colors yellow, blue, and green, but I don't like the color red. I just pretend that red doesn't exist. When I approach a red traffic light, what happens? I drive through and get injured in an accident, right? And because I can't see red, I wonder why I always get hurt through no fault of my own.

You wouldn't want to live a life where you didn't see red, would you? Even though they are all just colors, they are all equally important, all equally beautiful.

The same thing was happening to me with emotions. I was pretending to be positive only and ignoring the negative emotions. However, positive and negative emotions are just labels. In truth, emotions are emotions, and they are *all good*, they are all healthy to experience, and they all have their usefulness. The most commonly repressed emotions are anger and rage because they are not socially acceptable.

How do you deal with anger and rage?

This mislabeling of emotions as being positive and negative caused me to judge the negative ones and pretend they don't exist. As Adam Heller says, "The emotions that you don't give a voice to stay in your body as pain." Once I started to see emotions as analogous to colors, I no longer judged the ones I didn't want to feel. There are a lot of negative emotions in the two examples I listed above. Even though I didn't write any of them down in my journal, they were still there in my body. When I allow myself to feel my full spectrum of emotions, I am complete and multidimensional, and most important, I am also pain free.

Now that you have seen some examples of how only positivity can lead to repressed emotions, here are some examples of a few personality traits where a person may favor positivity and repress emotions:

A perfectionist may ignore negative emotions when things don't go perfectly. I am definitely 100 percent in this category. At Zero Pain Now* we've found that 80 percent of people suffering chronic pain are perfectionists. Be honest with this question: Are you a perfectionist?

The second largest category of personalities in pain are the spiritual or religious personalities. Usually a person with this personality type believes in seeing goodness and the positive side of everything. While this is wonderful, it makes it easy for this person to ignore negative emotions that tend to come up when parts of the world don't conform to the same spiritual ideal. And this person might not feel it's appropriate to acknowledge negative emotions. Can you relate to being spiritual or religious?

Some other personality traits conducive to emotional disconnection include those people who are "people pleasers," "do-gooders," or "controllers." I must confess I am *all* of these as well. What comes up when I'm unable to please someone? Or I see someone doing something "bad"? Or unable to control the outcome of something or to get someone to do what I want? Emotions, of course.

Can you relate to any of these personality types? Having even one of these is enough to cause you to be susceptible to disconnecting from your emotions and having DPS.

What's important to keep in mind is that there is no need to try to change your personality. Having chronic pain and becoming aware that you have some of the personality traits I've mentioned means you likely have a propensity to disconnect from those negative emotions. Once you recognize you have these characteristics, you can then allow yourself to connect to all the emotions, not just the positive, socially acceptable ones.

There have been many cases where people have become pain-free simply by becoming aware of their personality. I've helped people lower their pain levels just by allowing them to notice their personalities and then the emotions they weren't aware of—in one conversation.

You don't have to change being a perfectionist or any of the other personality types. For example, if you were an aircraft engineer, I'd want perfection in your product. You can't decide that a few inches here and there don't matter, otherwise the plane would crash. While perfection may be important in some aspects of our lives, it doesn't have to affect our ability to feel our emotions. The only thing you have to do is become aware of all your emotions, including those that may be generated by your personality type, especially the ones you tend to repress.

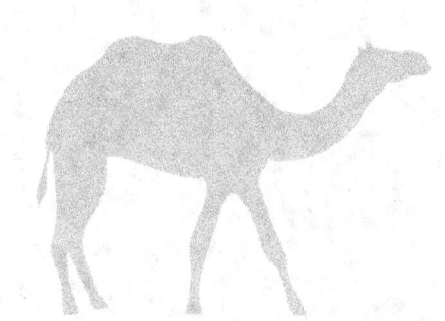

"Know thyself."

- Socrates

37
HOW DO YOU KNOW YOU ARE HEALED?

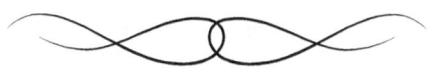

Each day I was pain-free was a feeling of joy, but the thought that kept coming up was, Maybe this is too good to be true. But after one month passed, then three months, six months, one year, two years, and more, I'm finally in my fifth year, and the pain has not returned. So I know with absolute certainty that the pain was caused by my disconnecting from certain emotions.

There have been moments when I feel a twinge or my back muscles getting tighter, and I just pause and inventory my emotions. I ask myself, "Right now, what emotion am I feeling?" I allow myself to feel whatever is coming up. And I'm often surprised at the emotions that pop up after I allow myself to feel them, emotions I was completely unaware of, and in an instant my muscles relax, with no further progression toward pain.

For instance, I once parked my car and paid the parking fee. As I walked off, I felt my back starting to tighten up. I then inventoried my emotions. Inventorying emotions is as simple as lowering your attention to your neck, chest, and belly area, and noticing what sensations are coming up, then labeling those sensations as emotions. When I did this I realized I was feeling angry. What about? The city had tripled the parking fees. I had just paid, so there was nothing I could do about it. I had initially blocked the emotion, but when I connected to it, the tightness immediately subsided. Of course, I didn't park there anymore, and I wrote to the city about the injustice of tripling the parking rate, both of which resulted in no change (and even more emotions!). But at least I was pain-free. It's important to feel the emotions even if they don't solve the immediate problem you are facing. But it definitely solves the immediate problem of risking having pain triggered.

As you may recall, dancing was something I thought I would do in another lifetime. So, after a year of being pain-free, I started taking dance classes, specifically salsa Casino style. As I would do the spins and turns, I was sure my pain would return. And for a few seconds I did feel the tightness. I connected to my emotions by tuning into my body and noticed that I felt fear. I acknowledged the fear and continued to dance. In a moment the muscle tightness was gone.

> **What do you dream of being able to do if you were pain-free right now?**

Dancing has been my ultimate healing. To know that I can dance, to twirl and spin and lead my partner while putting my body at its highest capability of movement, and to know that I can do it absolutely pain-free, was something I never could have imagined. After eight years of suffering it wasn't easy for me to forget the days of excruciating pain, and dancing is my greatest reminder that I am now pain-free and can live a normal life filled with smiles and doing the normal physical activities I always dreamed of doing.

I can help you get there with this book.

In the next few chapters I share stories of a few of the clients I have helped to get better. And after these I will expound on the healing process so you can get better and heal yourself too.

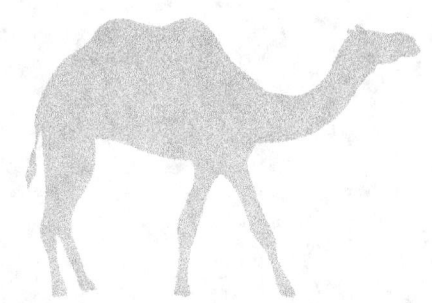

"I danced for three hours straight with no pain!"

- Mike

38
MIKE'S BACK PAIN

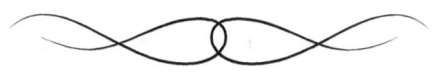

Mike was referred to me by his chiropractor, whom he had been going to for three years because of his back pain. Mike worked in construction, helping people remodel kitchens and bathrooms and create other home improvements.

He told me his pain began three years ago, and he attributed it to his construction work, which involved lifting and bending and a lot of physical labor. He would feel better after his chiropractic session, but his pain would return the next day. He was in so much pain that when he came home from work in the evening, he was hunched over, and all he could do was sit on his sofa and rest.

Before accepting him as a client, I asked him if he was open to the possibility that his pain was not a structural issue. He said, "It's not easy to believe, but yes, I'm open to that possibility." So I asked him to read *Zero Pain Now* by Adam Heller before we started the program. His initial pain level used to be an 11 out of 10 it was so high. Right after reading the book, his pain level dropped to a 5. He followed the book and companion workbook exactly as directed, and when we had his session on day 6, his pain started at a 3 and went down to zero.

For the next 22 days, Mike followed the instructions in the program and workbook exactly, and his pain stayed low. In the last week, it was down to zero and stayed there. He couldn't believe it. He asked himself, Is it gone? Is it really gone? Am I just not feeling it? Will it be back?

It didn't come back, and he completed the program completely pain-free and back to his full physical ability.

Now in the evenings, instead of lying on the sofa in pain, he goes out dancing. These are his exact words: "I was on the dance floor for three hours straight. *I'm not just doing dancing, I'm jumping around like a jumping bean!* And I'm 50 years old."

Nothing makes me happier than to see my clients living life at their full potential. Mike is still pain-free today, two years later, and continues to enjoy his physical activities to the maximum. The statement I loved most when I spoke to him last was, "There is nothing wrong with my back!"

"And you can't even carry more than one gallon of milk."

- Lisa

39
LISA'S NECK PAIN

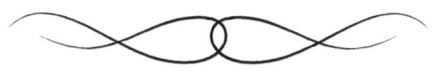

Lisa was a Zero Pain Now® client who had suffered more than 20 years of different kinds of pain. She had back and neck pain and was even diagnosed with fibromyalgia.

At times her back pain was extreme. She said, "When you can't sit down for three years in a row, and you can't even carry more than one gallon of milk in the house at a time when you used to carry televisions up two flights of stairs, you really know what it's like to be disabled from chronic pain."

She began the program focused on reducing her neck pain. She wanted to go backpacking with her husband, but because of the neck pain, for many years she had been unable to do so.

By the end of the 28-day program, not only was her back pain and neck pain down to zero, her firbromylagia symptoms were also gone.

Her one word to describe the program: "Shocking!"

"Life-changing."

- John

40
JOHN'S KNEE PAIN

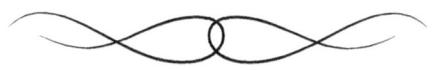

John was a client who came into the Zero Pain Now® program suffering from knee pain. He had knee surgery 11 years before, and after the surgery his knee became worse. He couldn't put any weight on it. You may recall the study I listed earlier which showed that fake knee surgeries showed just as much improvement as real knee surgeries.

He loved to play pickleball, and he was now limited at sports and other daily activities. Managing his pain by not putting any weight on his bad knee, he knew what his limitations were and avoided doing those things.

He too began the program by reading *Zero Pain Now*. His pain level was an 8 at the start of the program, and it dropped to a 5 after he read the book. By day 6 of the program his pain was down to level 1. He was delighted. However, in the next few days his pain level began to increase again. He realized he had to continue following the process exactly as described, otherwise his pain would return. After a few days his pain level started dropping again. By the last week of the program, he had zero pain and was out playing pickleball as much as he wanted to.

He admitted that he had celebrated too early in the process, and that the additional days and help from the coaches ingrained the process in his mind such that by the time he finished the program, the process was as effortless as walking.

Aside from playing pickleball, he now goes out for long walks, which weren't possible before, and he does whatever activities he wants without having to manage his knee pain.

His one word for the program: "Life-changing."

"Just allow yourself the possibility that this will work."

- Carla

41
CARLA'S BACK PAIN

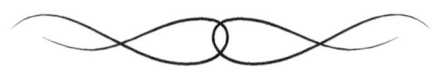

Carla suffered from back pain for many years. She was unable to bend, exercise, lift, lie down, stand up, or sit—"Just about anything," she said. "There was nowhere I could find comfort, and I was in a constant battle of managing my life around my pain." She tried stretching, yoga, medication, acupuncture, physical therapy, and chiropractic, which was her primary method because she was sure something must be out of place in her back.

She also was skeptical about healing from her pain when she started the program. The program seemed overly simplistic to her. How could pain be managed by words and thoughts?

But she followed the process diligently, and in 28 days she was pain-free or down to minimal pain. Her pain came back to level 3 on the last day of the program. After a call with her coaches, she was able to apply the process and bring the pain down to zero. This is completely normal because the new habits take some time to settle in. She has been pain-free ever since and described the program as "liberating." She is now able to pursue all her normal activities without any pain. In particular she can now resume her passion for yoga, weight lifting, and recumbent bike rides.

Her words: "Just allow yourself the possibility that this will work."

"I'm loading up bags of fertilizer and I have no pain."

- Israel

42
ISRAEL'S BACK PAIN

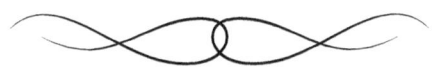

Israel was a client who came to the Zero Pain Now® program after 40 years of chronic back pain. He was the epitome of a person who has tried everything. He had several diagnoses, including stenosis, neuropathy, and degenerated disc disease. Over the years he had tried physical therapy, nerve ablations, injections, cauterizations, yoga, meditation, drugs, different kinds of chairs—almost everything possible, even more than I had.

Like Carla, he was skeptical of the Zero Pain Now® process and asked a lot of questions about the program. But most important, because he had tried so many structural healing modalities and had suffered so much, he was open to the possibility that his pain was not related to anything structural.

We began the program, and right away his pain dropped by several points. By day 10 he started to notice a significant difference in his pain level and realized the process was working. He was convinced. For the remaining 18 days, he followed the process to a tee and felt his pain drop to zero during the last week of the program.

He loved gardening, and at the end of the program he said, "I went to Home Depot, and I was loading up bags of fertilizer and had no pain. And I helped someone move furniture the other day and there was no pain." His 40 years of pain were gone in less than 28 days, and he was delighted. He is an inspiration to me because he is 70 years old, and I look forward to being as physical as he is when I'm 70.

"I can have sex without pain."

- Carlos

43
CARLOS'S UNDIAGNOSABLE BACK PAIN

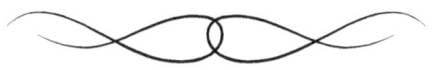

Carlos came into the Zero Pain Now® program suffering from back pain. He was referred to us by his healthcare providers. Six years ago he felt a stabbing pain in his back when he had done some heavy lifting. Since that day, his pain kept coming back.

Unlike the other clients described above, MRI scans showed nothing abnormal in his back. He had been suffering for many years and had seen many different doctors and specialists for his pain. But nothing was working. He was a young man who, prior to his pain, had been physically active, playing basketball and other team sports.

To manage the pain, he would get yearly nerve cauterizations. However, these cauterizations, also called ablations, would only last six months, and then he was in pain again. Even after the ablations, he was still at a physical ability level of 5, unable to play basketball and other sports he loved. He didn't want to continue doing the cauterizations; he wanted permanent relief.

When he started the program, he was at a pain level of 8 and a physical ability level of 3. Within the first six days, he followed the steps of the program exactly as written, and his pain level dropped to a 2. He soon started doing things around the house—gardening, fixing things, and working on his cars. By the end of the program he was completely pain-free and at full physical ability. At his exit interview the most memorable statement from him was that "I can have sex with my wife without pain."

"We don't laugh because we're happy—we're happy because we laugh."

- *William James, father of American psychology, 1842*

44
HOW YOU CAN HEAL YOURSELF

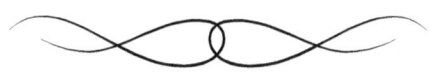

Now that you have seen how I healed myself as well as the success of several clients who followed the Zero Pain Now® program, you have the knowledge to heal yourself too.

As I mentioned at the beginning of this book, your story may not be the same, your symptoms may not be the same, your diagnosis may not be the same, but if you can *relate to my story of pain,* that's all that matters for you to heal yourself.

Regardless of your symptoms or diagnosis, were you able to relate to my story? Was your experience similar to mine? Are you being tossed around in the medical system with test after test and diagnosis after diagnosis without any personal attention? Have you noticed different answers and recommendations and diagnoses being provided for your pain? Have you found that something worked for a short while and then stopped working? Is it hard for you to let go of one modality and switch to another? Did you feel betrayed when something you were sure would work didn't? Are you frustrated with all the advice your friends, family, and others give you? Are you overwhelmed when you search on Google and see the number of solutions that are out there? Is your experience like having an invisible illness? Have you been told that you needed to come back for more treatments over and over again for some modality? Or have you been told that nothing can be done for your diagnosis?

If you have even one or two of these experiences, there is a very good chance that you can get better from any of the following symptoms or diagnoses:

Pain in the back, neck, shoulder, sciatic nerve, hip, knee, or foot, or migraines, TMJ (temporomandibular joint), whiplash, fibromyalgia, CRPS (Complex Regional Pain Syndrome), herniated disc, bulging disc, spinal stenosis, scoliosis, degenerative disc disease, neuropathy, tendonitis, carpal tunnel syndrome, spondylosis, spondylitis, plantar fasciitis, torn rotator cuff, torn meniscus, osteoarthritis-related pain, bone spurs, undiagnosable pain, and more.

If you can relate to my story, you have a good chance of healing yourself, because it is likely you have Diversion Pain Syndrome. If the wrong message is sent from the brain, an infinite number of symptoms can arise, combinations of pain, burning, tingling, numbness and weakness in various parts of your body. Just imagine the chaos at a traffic light that is receiving the wrong message. Doctors can spend lifetimes categorizing and diagnosing and treating these symptoms and doing research because, for them, this is exciting to study. But for you—you will still remain in pain.

The usual suspects are lined up, but they all have alibis. There is no proof beyond a reasonable doubt that they did the crime. If there was, we would all get better. Many of the usual suspects are a normal sign of aging. Bulging discs, herniated discs, osteoarthritis—these are all normal signs of aging and rarely cause pain. As Adam Heller says, "Getting surgery for normal signs of aging is like getting surgery for gray hair."

After the age of 50, according to the *American Journal of Radiology*, 80 percent of people have disc degeneration issues and are asymptomatic.[29] If degeneration contributed to pain, 80 percent of the people over 50 should be in chronic pain, but they aren't. Chronic pain is spread across all ages and is increasingly getting to the younger ages because they too are experiencing more stress and tension and a disconnection from certain emotions.

I have given you all the information required to heal yourself. Some people can get better just by reading this book. If this works for you, that's great. I also recommend rereading this book. I've emphasized certain sentences that are important for the healing process and will allow you to reread the book faster and with deeper meaning.

Are you ready to end your pain? Here are the simple steps to healing:

First, make sure you are checked out by a doctor to rule out any cancer or organic disease. Inform your doctor that you are doing a mind-body connection approach to healing. Now, take some time to journal about what was going on in your life around the time that your pain began.

For the next 30 days:

1. Acknowledge that the pain is not due to a structural abnormality in your body. Your body and its systems are fine and healthy.

2. The reason for the pain is a reduction in blood flow leading to a mild oxygen deprivation triggered by a disconnection from certain repressed emotions.

3. Inventory your life *right now* and look at everything going on, especially things you might not want to confront. Make a list of items adding stress to your life. Make a new list each day. On the first day, write down at least one hundred items.

4. Journal for about 30 minutes on the items on this list.

5. For at least 15 minutes nonstop every day, ask yourself this question: "Right now what emotion am I feeling?" Ask this question out loud. Then answer out loud to yourself, "I am feeling _____," filling in an emotion. Write down your one-word answer each time on a piece of paper. Repeat until you are able to empty out all your emotions by simply acknowledging them. Repeat as needed throughout the day.

6. The emotions have no meaning; they are just like the colors of a rainbow—all good and normal to feel. Pay most attention to feeling your "negative" emotions. A tip: Negative emotions tend to reside as sensations in the neck, chest, and belly area. Just notice these sensations and label them as emotions. Research has shown we experience a feeling a split second before we can intellectualize about it.[30]

7. Think psychological, not physical. The pain is a symptom. The pain is not an emotion. Notice and label your emotions, not the pain.

8. Notice your personality traits and be aware of how they contribute to generating emotions and possibly repressing emotions. Journal on these traits if needed.

9. Daily increase your physical activities as you are able to—until you can return to normal, regular activity. Increasing your activity is critical to healing because it proves to you that you do not have a structural issue. The pain is a symptom. The pain is not an emotion. Notice and label your emotions, not the pain.

10. Use these tools for the rest of your life, and you'll stay pain-free.

Remember, the repressed emotions are usually about things that you have no control over and that conflict with your self-image, which can be a good reason to not want to feel them. Acknowledge that they are just emotions, with no more meaning to them than that.

This process can be done daily as needed until you have completely healed yourself and built a habit of automatically connecting to your emotions as effortlessly as walking. If you do this conscientiously for 30 days, this new way of processing emotions will become automatic.

Your success is measured as:

- Little or no more pain
- Back to normal physical ability
- No more drugs or pain management tools
- No more fear

"Great is the man who has not lost his childlike heart."

- Mencius

45
FINAL WORDS

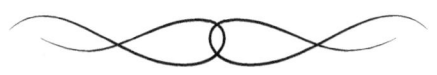

While it might not be easy to believe this solution works, believe me when I say I have been pain-free for five years. I have noticed that my pain returns sometimes, but in a matter of minutes I can banish it by connecting to emotions about something going on in my life. It's as simple as that. And this is how I know that this solution is not a placebo but instead addresses the cause of the pain directly. And thousands of Zero Pain Now® clients are permanently pain-free with this understanding of the origin and cause of the pain.

Added benefits for me have been no more headaches, and even my seasonal allergies are gone and I sleep much better at night. Think of a backache as just like a headache, only in the back. When you get a headache, you don't think of structural issues. It just goes away on its own. A backache can do the same thing if you don't think of it as a structural issue.

Do you suffer from headaches, gastrointestinal issues, and insomnia?

We have found that 80 percent of chronic pain sufferers also suffer from headaches and gastrointestinal issues, which usually clear up after healing from the pain.

The Straw That Broke the Camel's Back

There will always be stress and tension in our lives. This is what living means. We all have finances, significant others, family, in-laws, house payments, car payments, bosses, clients, and a multitude of things adding stress to our lives. If a dozen or more of these are not affecting you daily, then you probably live alone on a mountain top and meditate deeply all day long. The way to manage the stress is to allow yourself to recognize all the emotions and let them pass through, because they are just like a warning light in our car. We acknowledge the warning and then take whatever actions are needed.

Our emotions are part our signaling network. The saying "the straw that broke the camel's back" describes this perfectly: the seemingly minor or routine action that causes an unpredictably large and sudden reaction because of the cumulative effect of small actions. A small message from the brain can make a small change in the body by reducing blood flow, which reduces oxygen, and this results in pain, burning, tingling, numbness, or weakness, with all kinds of symptoms and often excruciating pain. Change the signal and the pain stops.

Thanks to my experiences and pain-free existence, I'm now a better swimmer, and I have a good knowledge of anatomy and know how to maintain a good posture. I may even take up yoga, though it never was very appealing to me. And of course, I am now a dancer, which still makes me smile because that was not something I ever imagined myself doing. I also no longer dream about muscle and spinal transplants, though I do hope they happen before AD 2364 in the genuine cases where they are required! Medicine is amazing, and I am a fan when it is truly needed.

But more than anything, I'm grateful that I've been able to help hundreds of people learn how to become pain-free after all hope has been taken away from them. A client recently emailed me a picture of her walking cane. "I don't need this anymore!" she said after her pain was gone. This gives me the greatest joy in life.

I'm going to close with another of my favorite quotes from a famous psychologist and the founder of gestalt therapy:

> Lose Your Mind and Come to Your Senses
> **Fritz Perls**

I want to reiterate that the information in this book is not to replace medical advice. I only see clients with a medical referral from a licensed practitioner. Medicine is marvelous and amazing and capable of magnificent miracles. I only help in those situations where medicine is able to treat the symptoms but not the cause of pain.

You now know and understand the straw that breaks your back, or whatever diagnosis you have been given. It's not your fault. Like Sherlock Holmes said, once you eliminate the impossible, whatever remains, no matter how improbable, must be the truth. By building a habit of noticing the sensations in your neck, chest, and belly area, and by labeling them out loud as emotions, you can stop the straw that keeps breaking your back (or other part of your body that is in pain). You can heal yourself and get back your freedom and independence. I wish you a wonderful and pain-free life.

Love,
Brajesh

"If there's no meaning in it," said the King, "that saves a world of trouble, you know, as we needn't try to find any."

- *Lewis Caroll, Alice in Wonderland*

FREQUENTLY ASKED QUESTIONS

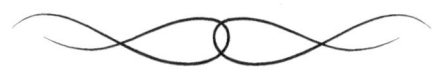

1. **Do I have to change my personality to become pain-free?**

   Absolutely not. Your personality is what gives you your success in life. You simply need to become aware of the emotions your personality can generate.

2. **Do I have to become a more emotional person?**

   No. Nothing outward changes. Your friends will probably not notice anything different about you. The emotions only need to be felt and acknowledged internally.

3. **Do I have to become outgoing and extroverted?**

   No. Nothing outward changes. No actions are necessary.

4. **Do I have to do anything when I feel my emotions?**

   Absolutely not. Just allow yourself to feel and acknowledge them. There's no meaning to the emotions. That's all that's needed to get you to be pain-free. It's as easy as lying in a hammock and relaxing. You are safe.

5. **Are there other benefits of this solution?**

    Yes, many, and these vary with clients. Almost all Zero Pain Now® clients have reported becoming more assertive in their lives. Many have improved their sleep. Some have reduced or almost eliminated their allergies. Many no longer have gastrointestinal issues or headaches.

6. **How do I know this method will work for me?**

    First, check with your doctor to see if you can undergo such a program, and to make sure he or she has ruled out cancer and any organic disease. Next you can take a pain test that will tell you with 95 percent certainty whether you have Diversion Pain Syndrome or not:

    www.paintest.org

    Realize that most of the diagnoses mentioned in this book are normal signs of aging where many people in the population have structural defects but no pain. And if you have no structural defects, like Carlos's example, you are in an even better place.

7. **Why would I take the Zero Pain Now® program when I have this book?**

    Some people may need some additional guided help, and I can help you to get yourself pain-free through the licensed Zero Pain Now® coaching program. In this program you will have a private coach to guide you daily until you are pain-free.

8. **Can positive events generate stress and tension?**

   Absolutely. A marriage, a new baby, a promotion—all are events that cause a change and can generate stress and tension. Any event that causes a *change*, whether positive or negative, will generate stress and tension.

9. **What chronic conditions do not qualify for this process?**

   Any kind of cancer. Multiple sclerosis. Rheumatoid arthritis. Any kind of organic illness. Always check with your doctor first and get their approval before taking on this program.

10. **If I pay attention to my negative emotions, will I become a negative person?**

    While this may apply to many things in life, when it comes to emotions, this is a common misconception. Frequent research has shown the exact opposite effect. Putting feelings into words, or the process of "affect labeling," can diffuse the negative emotions and enhance the positive emotions. It's a win-win for you to notice all your emotions! [31]

> Putting feelings into words, or "affect labeling," can attenuate our emotional experiences.
>
> **"Emotion Review" journal**

11. **I sometimes suppress my emotions. Is that the same thing as repression?**

    No. Emotions you know about are not the ones causing pain. Repression by definition means something you are unaware of. Thinking, Fast and Slow by Nobel laureate and psychologist Daniel Kahneman is an excellent book that describes how automatic and invisible our mind is. He summarizes the concept perfectly by this statement: "You know less about yourself than you think you do."

12. **What are the common emotions keeping me in pain?**

    The most common emotions contributing to pain are anger, rage, hurt, sadness, fear, guilt, shame, jealousy, disgust, anxiety, resentment, disappointment, frustration, worry, exasperation, disgust, irritation, panic, envy, overwhelm, and feeling harassed, embarrassed, or annoyed.

ACKNOWLEDGMENTS

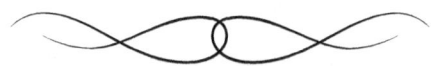

Several people have helped me on my journey to becoming pain-free. I would like to express my gratitude to all of them for improving the quality of my life:

- My friend Amit who introduced me to the process of healing myself.

- Dr. John O'Connell, my first doctor, who told me everything I needed to know, and I didn't understand it.

- Dr. Mark D. Brown, who reassured me that I was structurally fine.

- Kristin, my physical therapist who always took away my pain every time I went to see her.

- My parents, who stayed by me throughout my pain, never judging me for not being able to help them lift things.

- Gloria, for bringing me groceries when I had my first episode.

- Nastasia and Patricia, for taking care of my sitting needs wherever we went.

- My brother Sanjay, for spending three weeks with me when I had my first episode, and helping me get back on my feet.

- Dr. Hajera Fatima, who kept encouraging me to find the root cause of my chronic pain.

- Ankush Jain, who coached me to keep going even when I wasn't getting results.

- Jeff Braucher, my editor who painstakingly read my manuscript and made it clear, concise, and consistent.

- Karen Bomm, my author strategist. Without her meticulous guidance I could never publish this book.

- Dan Buglio and Matthew Rosett for guiding me to the next steps to that allowed me to master step 2.

- Adam Heller, for creating the amazing process that got me pain-free in a matter of days and whose simple process has kept me pain-free.

REFERENCES

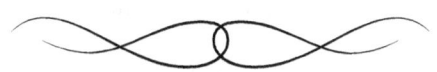

1   Ethics - Star Trek the Next Generation, 1992, Season 5, Episode 16

2   Boston University School of Public Health, Chronic Pain and the Health of Populations, Sandro Galea, MD and Goldberg DS, McGee SJ. Pain as a global public health priority. BMC Public Health. 2011 Oct 6;11:770. doi: 10.1186/1471-2458-11-770. PMID: 21978149; PMCID: PMC3201926.

3   https://en.wikipedia.org/wiki/Straw_that_broke_the_camel's_back

4   *The Sign of the Four,* Sir Arthur Conan Doyle

5   Fatoye, F., Gebrye, T. & Odeyemi, I. Real-world incidence and prevalence of low back pain using routinely collected data. Rheumatol Int 39, 619–626 (2019). https://doi.org/10.1007/s00296-019-04273-0

6   Brox, Jens Ivar. "Lifting with straight legs and bent spine is not bad for your back" *Scandinavian Journal of Pain*, vol. 18, no. 4, 2018, pp. 563-564. https://doi.org/10.1515/sjpain-2018-0302

7   From a study in the *American Journal of Sports Medicine*, April 2007. Article in the *Chicago Tribune*, Former NFL players live with pain, by Sandra G. Boodman. https://www.chicagotribune.com/news/ct-xpm-2007-05-15-0705130303-story.html

8   Agassi, A. (2010). *Open*. HarperCollins.

9   Occupational Safety and Health Administration. osha.gov

10 https://www.businessinsider.com/moderna-designed-coronavirus-vaccine-in-2-days-2020-11

11 *N Engl J Med* 1994; 331:69-73 DOI: 10.1056/NEJM199407143310201, https://www.nejm.org/doi/full/10.1056/NEJM199407143310201

12 Sarno MD, John, *Healing Back Pain: The Mind-Body Connection*, Warner Books

13 Baber Z, Erdek MA. Failed back surgery syndrome: current perspectives. *J Pain Res*. 2016;9:979-987. Published 2016 Nov 7. doi:10.2147/JPR.S92776

14 Kordi R, Rostami M. Low back pain in children and adolescents: an algorithmic clinical approach. *Iran J Pediatr*. 2011;21(3):259-270.

15 https://www.drugabuse.gov/drug-topics/opioids/opioid-overdose-crisis

16 https://www.cdc.gov/media/releases/2020/p1218-overdose-deaths-covid-19.html

17 Freburger JK, Holmes GM, Agans RP, et al. The rising prevalence of chronic low back pain. *Arch Intern Med*. 2009;169(3):251-258. doi:10.1001/

archinternmed.2008.543 https://www.ncbi.nlm.nih.gov/pmc/articles/PMC4339077/

18   https://en.wikipedia.org/wiki/The_Invitation, Seinfeld, 1996

19   *N Engl J Med* 2002; 347:81-88 DOI: 10.1056/NEJMoa013259 https://www.nejm.org/doi/full/10.1056/NEJMoa013259

20   https://www.washingtonpost.com/health/opioid-settlement-drug-distributors/2020/11/05/6a8da214-1fc7-11eb-b532-05c751cd5dc2_story.html

21   Gaskin DJ, Richard P. The Economic Costs of Pain in the United States. In: Institute of Medicine (US) Committee on Advancing Pain Research, Care, and Education. *Relieving Pain in America: A Blueprint for Transforming Prevention, Care, Education, and Research.* Washington (DC): National Academies Press (US); 2011. Appendix C. Available from: https://www.ncbi.nlm.nih.gov/books/NBK92521/

22   Rosomoff, H. L. "Presentation at the American Academy of Pain Medicine 17th Annual Meeting." Miami, Florida (2001).

23   Lucas AJ. Failed back surgery syndrome: whose failure? Time to discard a redundant term. *British Journal of Pain.* 2012;6(4):162-165. doi:10.1177/2049463712466517

24   Shipton EE, Bate F, Garrick R, Steketee C, Shipton EA, Visser EJ. Systematic Review of Pain Medicine Content, Teaching, and Assessment in Medical School Curricula Internationally. *Pain Ther.* 2018;7(2):139-161. doi:10.1007/s40122-018-0103-z

25 Lund N, Bengtsson A, Thorborg P. Muscle tissue oxygen pressure in primary fibromyalgia. *Scand J Rheumatol.* 1986;15(2):165-73. doi: 10.3109/03009748609102084. PMID: 3462905.

https://www.ncbi.nlm.nih.gov/pubmed/3462905

26 https://en.wikipedia.org/wiki/Classical_conditioning

27 Emma Young, July 2018, New Scientist.

Leonard Mlodinow, Subliminal—How Your Unconscious Mind Rules Your Behavior - Pantheon Books 2012, p34.

28 Gatchel, Robert J., Peng, Yuan Bo, Peters, Madelon L.; Fuchs, Perry N.; Turk, Dennis C. 2007 The biopsychosocial approach to chronic pain: Scientific advances and future directions *Psychological Bulletin*, Vol 133(4), 581-624

29 W. Brinjikji, P.H. Luetmer, B. Comstock, B.W. Bresnahan, L.E. Chen, R.A. Deyo, S. Halabi, J.A. Turner, A.L. Avins, K. James, J.T. Wald, D.F. Kallmes and J.G. Jarvik.

American Journal of Neuroradiology, April 2015, 36 (4) 811-816; DOI: https://doi.org/10.3174/ajnr.A4173 http://www.ajnr.org/content/36/4/8116

30 Zajonc, R. B. (1980). Feeling and thinking: Preferences need no inferences. American Psychologist, 35(2), 151–175. https://doi.org/10.1037/0003-066X.35.2.151

31 Torre JB, Lieberman MD. Putting Feelings Into Words: Affect Labeling as Implicit Emotion Regulation. *Emotion Review*. 2018;10(2):116-124. doi:10.1177/175407391774270

ABOUT THE AUTHOR

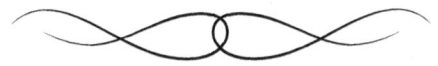

Brajesh K. Singh has a Master of Science in Computer Engineering.

He has over 20 years' experience designing communication networks.

Starting in 2009, he endured eight years of chronic back pain. Using his engineering mindset, he attempted to methodically solve his pain. Over eight years he found many ways that didn't work, and he was stuck with managing his pain until finally he discovered the Zero Pain Now® solution that ended his pain permanently.

He was surprised to discover the connection between communication networks and the communications network of the human nervous system. The health of a communications network and the human nervous system is the content of its messages.

Brajesh is a certified Zero Pain Now® Master Coach.

CONNECT WITH ME

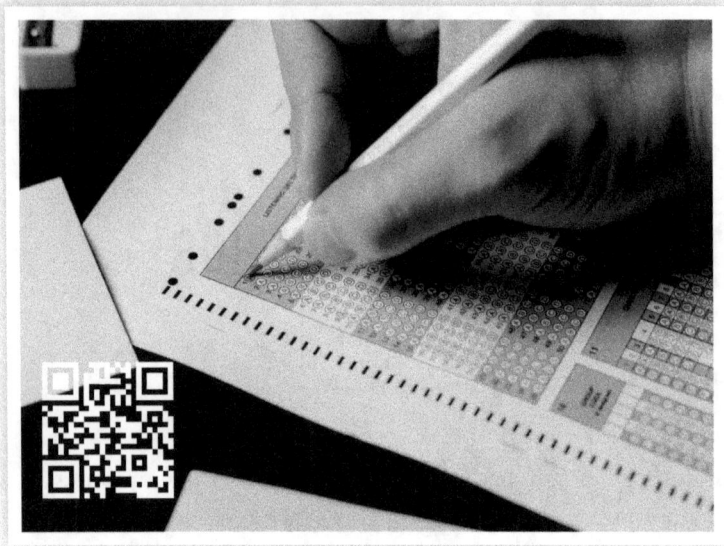

Take this 2 minute online pain test to determine
if you have Diversion Pain Syndrome.

Discover my online programs
to help you heal yourself.

CONNECT WITH ME

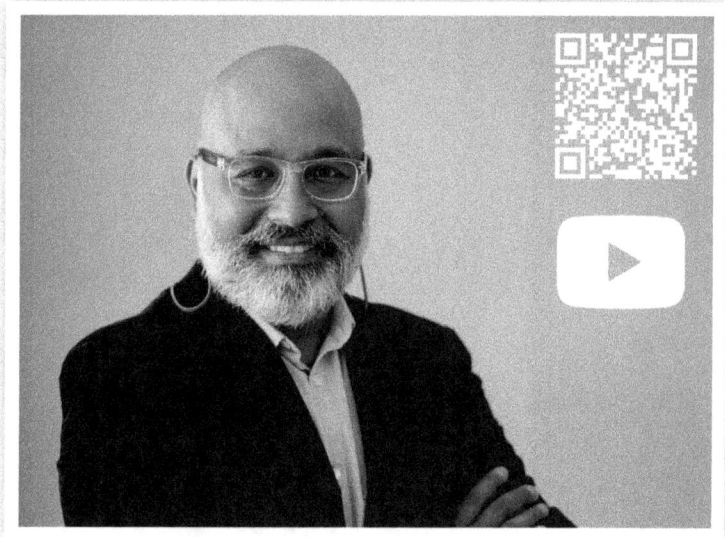

Subscribe to my YouTube videos and
watch my content to help you heal yourself.

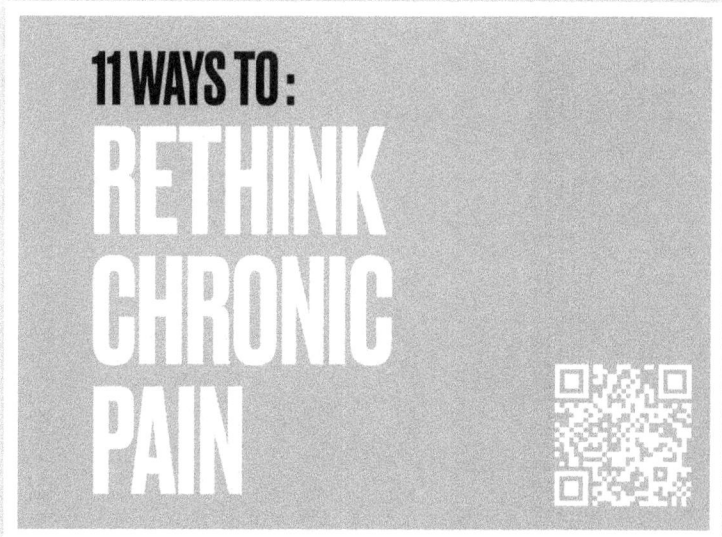

Download my free ebook and
get additional tips to heal yourself.

www.ingramcontent.com/pod-product-compliance
Lightning Source LLC
LaVergne TN
LVHW011825060526
838200LV00053B/3899